Praise for *Saying Yes*

"Few books capture the real, lived experience of opening a relationship with such honesty and heart. In *Saying Yes,* Natalie Davis invites us into the raw, beautiful, and sometimes messy process of navigating love, jealousy, desire, and growth outside traditional norms. With refreshing candor and courage, she illuminates the longing, uncertainty, joy, and heartbreak that can arise along the way. For anyone curious about consensual non-monogamy or seeking to better understand their own relationship landscape, this book is a generous and affirming companion."

—Jessica Fern, author of *Polysecure, Polywise,* and *Transforming the Shame Triangle*

"This memoir is witty, refreshingly honest, and deeply relatable. Natalie's voice is endearing without ever turning saccharine, offering a vulnerable and candid exploration of polyamory with all its trials, tribulations, and hard-earned triumphs. The result is a thoughtful and often humorous portrait of love, identity, and connection, told through the many ups and downs of real life."

—Kate Kincaid, LPC, author of *Polyamory Journal*

"*Saying Yes* is a brutally honest and beautifully rendered account of how one happily married couple chose to expand their love into a polyamory lifestyle. Natalie Davis shows every vulnerable, humorous, and challenging aspect of this choice, all while educating 'normies' with pertinent terminology and sharing her deepest feelings, fears, failures, and triumphs. The sincerity, earnestness, and authenticity of their journey had me entranced from the very first page. This book is not to be missed!"

—Lorelei James, *New York Times* bestselling author

"Many twenty-first-century couples will see themselves in the author's story: Her queasy entry into swinging at her husband's urging, her experience with a disastrous first metamour, and the couple's slow advance into full, loving, community-centric polyamory. We learn from experience, but it's a lot less painful to learn from other people's experiences. Any couple thinking about consensual non-monogamy can learn a lot from reading and discussing this book."

—Alan MacRobert, *Polyamory in the News*

"This unflinchingly honest memoir lays bare one woman's exploration of consensual non-monogamy and polyamory. In the tone of your wise best friend, Natalie Davis blends intimate life stories with practical information, including a much-needed legal perspective and a spotlight on the challenges and importance of finding a poly-affirming therapist. *Saying Yes* is an insightful read for anyone new to navigating a mix of love, sex, marriage, and non-monogamy."

—Tamara Pincus, co-author of *It's Called "Polyamory"*

"Through vivid and vulnerable storytelling, Natalie Davis offers the kind of authentic polyamory narrative that builds understanding and breaks down barriers."

—Brett Chamberlin, Executive Director of OPEN

"One of my favorite things about polyamory is how different our journeys all are. Like Natalie, I started my polyamorous adventure with my college sweetheart. But while the rest of our paths diverged wildly, we both experienced wins and losses that shaped our lives in unbelievable ways. *Saying Yes* not only gives insight on the highs and lows of polyamory, but from the very title it reminds us of the value of giving yourself permission and putting yourself out there. Dating, relationships, love, and life don't have to be perfect to be worth celebrating."

—Kevin Patterson, creator of Poly Role Models and author of *Love's Not Colorblind*

"I've had the pleasure of meeting Natalie several times, and her genuine no-nonsense approach to sharing her story is exactly what comes through in *Saying Yes*. She doesn't sugarcoat the messy, complicated reality of navigating polyamory—she tells it like it is, mistakes and all, which is exactly what people need to hear when they're considering their own authentic path. If you're curious about polyamory or just want to read about someone's brave journey toward living authentically, this memoir offers the raw honesty and real-world perspective that's often missing from relationship advice."

—Kitty Chambliss, MCC, CPC, TIC, author of *Jealousy Survival Guide*

SAYING YES

SAYING YES

My Adventures in Polyamory

Natalie Davis

Skyhorse Publishing

Skyhorse Publishing books may be purchased in bulk at special discounts for sales promotion, corporate gifts, fund-raising, or educational purposes. Special editions can also be created to specifications. For details, contact the Special Sales Department, Skyhorse Publishing, 307 West 36th Street, 11th Floor, New York, NY 10018 or info@skyhorsepublishing.com.

Skyhorse® and Skyhorse Publishing® are registered trademarks of Skyhorse Publishing, Inc.®, a Delaware corporation.

Visit our website at www.skyhorsepublishing.com.

Please follow our publisher Tony Lyons on Instagram @tonylyonsisuncertain.

10 9 8 7 6 5 4 3 2 1

Library of Congress Cataloging-in-Publication Data is available on file.

Cover design by David Ter-Avanesyan

Print ISBN: 978-1-5107-8449-9
Ebook ISBN: 978-1-5107-8451-2

Printed in the United States of America

For RtM

Gratitude

I am beyond grateful to the polyamorous and poly-friendly folks who have contributed to this book by serving as inspirations, sounding boards, editors, lovers, dear friends, and, in the best-case scenario, all of the above. You make my heart sing.

In September 2006, the Oxford English Dictionary added an entry for *polyamory*:

> The fact of having simultaneous close emotional relationships with two or more other individuals, viewed as an alternative to monogamy, esp. in regard to matters of sexual fidelity; the custom or practice of engaging in multiple sexual relationships with the knowledge and consent of all partners concerned.

***

Ask for what you want. Be prepared to hear "no."

—Paraphrase of poly wisdom derived from
What Did I Learn Today? Lessons on the Journey to Self-Love
by Akosua Dardaine Edwards (2013)

Contents

PART THREE

Author's Note

This book is based on true events. It reflects my present recollections of experiences over time, aided by conversations with participants and my contemporaneous records, including emails, texts, and notes. All names and some characteristics have been changed, some events have been compressed, and some dialogue has been recreated. This was done to protect the privacy of individuals and for narrative purposes.

Preface

Welcome to my polyamorous life. I have been some flavor of non-monogamous for more than twenty-five years and have identified as polyamorous since 2010. For me, being polyamorous means having intimate relationships independent of my husband. Polyamory is a form of consensual non-monogamy where everyone involved has agreed to the relationship structure and to be open and honest.

Eric and I fell in love in college. We were in a traditional, committed, monogamous relationship for more than ten years, before and after marriage and parenthood. I was raised by loving parents, who were together until cancer stole my mother. My engineer father was the first feminist I knew, and my artist mother's mantra to her two daughters was "Don't marry a doctor or a lawyer; be one," and I listened. I cheered for my first-baseman sister from the Little League snack stand, not minding that my arms were sticky up to the elbows from handing out snow cones.

Eric and I have lived and worked in the Washington, DC, area for most of our adult lives. We have volunteered in our community and traded pet-sitting favors with our neighbors. I used to say our tattoo count was zero, but Eric finally got inked with an infinity symbol encircling a robust heart—the polyamory emblem.

We frequent rock concerts and dance to gothic, industrial, synthpop, darkwave, and '80s pop music at clubs and in our living room under the disco light Eric installed for me as a surprise birthday present. We have hosted our friends for cookouts and a quarterly benevolent dictatorship and feed fest named Natalie's Book Club. Our closets are mostly black. Mine has dashes of crimson and fuchsia, and even a few floral patterns. Don't tell my goth friends about the flowered dresses.

And yes, Eric and I are poly—short for polyamorous. We date other people. We have sex with other people. We have intimate relationships with other people. And, if we are fortunate, we love other people. I think it's terrific. I did not start out thinking that way, but now I do. I am no expert with a fancy degree, but I have twenty-five years of personal experience with non-monogamy, both ethical and not. I have screwed up—and just screwed—since boarding the poly ship. My practice of polyamory has changed, and I hope it has improved.

For those considering some form of non-monogamy and those who have already dipped their toes into the waters, I want you to know that you are not alone. For those simply curious about this crazy thing called polyamory—it's in the news, in the courts, and probably in your neighborhood—why not take a peek?

Natalie Davis
nataliedavisadventures.com

SAYING YES

PART ONE

1.

Origin Story

I awoke to the rich aroma of coffee brewing downstairs and turned to face the clock on the nightstand. At a little after ten on a Sunday morning, there was just enough time before my gym class for a quick bite and, yes, coffee. My husband was making breakfast. Breakfast à la Eric was scrambled eggs, a bagel with cream cheese and lox, lightly pulped orange juice, and sugary instant cinnamon-flavored coffee from a tin. The drip coffee was for me, prepared by my husband's girlfriend. She brewed it stronger than I did, but I liked it. I especially liked that it was being made for me while I slept in the spare room.

I leaned sideways in the bed. "Babe," I whispered to my lover, "Eric is making breakfast. Are you hungry?"

* * *

Ten years into our marriage, Eric said, "I know what I want for my birthday."

Eric and I met in college. He was a skinny twenty-year old with dark hair. Just shy of six feet tall, he wore large, round, black-framed glasses, typical of the 1980s. In the seventeen years that had brought us to that day, before and after marriage and the birth of our son, I had always agonized over what to get Eric for his birthday.

"Oh yeah?' I asked. "What?"

"I'm going to pull up a website. Please keep an open mind and read it all. Then we can talk about it."

I looked at my husband. In his mid-thirties then, Eric was still slender, but after becoming a dedicated gym member, he had achieved a more muscular build. That mattered to him. I liked the way he looked and the way he felt against me, with or without the harder pecs. Neither of us had changed much since college. I wore my straight, dark hair in a short bob rather than the midback-length style I had sported when Eric and I met. I had lobbed my locks soon after we started dating because, at nineteen, I yearned to look older. Eric was short-haired and clean-shaven, as befitted the National Guardsman he had been since he was seventeen. He had recently made the Army his full-time career in a headquarters posting.

I was still within a respectable distance of my college sophomore figure. Eric's roommate had teased him that we looked disturbingly like siblings with our dark hair and eyes, generous noses, and similar body types. A dozen years after we met, it was no surprise that our son Will was born long and lanky with such deep brown eyes that you had to look closely to discern his pupils. No mischievous blond Calvin for us, even though our looks mirrored those of his comic strip parents, and one of Will's favorite stuffed animals was a floppy striped tiger.

The website for "The Lodge" listed no physical address. The home page advised that directions would be provided after signing in. I raised an eyebrow and read on. There was a dance floor, buffet, bar, pool tables, and private and group rooms. Rules were listed. *No means no. Always ask permission.* What?

You guessed it, or maybe not, because it certainly took me a moment. The Lodge was a nightclub for swingers, a term that made me cringe. "Lifestyle club" was the alternative lingo. From what I understood about such places—from movies, I supposed—couples, who might or might not already know each other, swapped partners and had sex.

The site was low-key. It had FAQs and photos of the club. My brow may have been knitted, but I was still reading. "Okay," I said, sighing only slightly. "I finished reading." I swiveled slowly on the desk chair and looked at Eric, my arms crossed over my chest. *This should be good.*

"I'd like to try this," he said. "We don't have to do anything other than check it out, but I'm curious." He spoke slowly and deliberately as if to avoid spooking a skittish colt. "I realize this is new, but I ask that you try to keep an open mind. That's all."

I felt my face redden and my heartbeat quicken. I was fighting off anger, not successfully. "Strangers hook up and swap partners in the middle of nowhere at someplace called The Lodge? That's what you want to do on your birthday? And you want me to do it with you? Seriously?" I groaned. "Eric . . . I don't know. . . ." Eric waited.

I was quiet, thinking. Eight months earlier, Eric had had an affair. As far as I knew, it was the first time he had cheated. Will had been a toddler. Eric's business had been struggling, and I had just lost my job. Eric's only income for months had been his three-way cut of the five-bucks-a-head door charge at a weekly goth club he promoted. That's where he met Katrina. *That slut with the bad haircut* was how I referred to her in my head when I learned, after Eric answered each question in my cross-examination—the consequence of marrying a lawyer—that he was not her first rodeo with a married man.

While job hunting on our shared computer, I had happened on an email from her, carelessly left open. Shaking with hurt, anger, and above all, humiliation, I called Eric at work. "I saw the email. Do you think I'm stupid?" I had hung up and paced, considering my options. Eric had rushed home.

I witnessed Eric crying for the first time. Over the next weeks, we talked a lot. We each found new jobs within a month. There were a lot of transitions for us as individuals and as a couple. We were still recovering the summer Eric made his birthday proposal.

Eric had risked his family for the validation he found in Katrina's bed. I was not fool enough to believe his needs had evaporated when the affair ended. I viewed Eric's openness in proposing this exploration with me as better than cheating. When we talked about his affair, Eric had said that the lying had torn him up.

Oh, poor baby. Was that hard for you? Shall I weep for your angst and your struggle?

"I hated lying to you. I felt dirty and knew you deserved better than that," he had said. "In my mind—perhaps it was just a fantasy—I had hoped that somehow this could have worked out, that you would see what I saw in Katrina and that you would have been friends because, although I know that you don't want to hear this now, you two have a lot in common."

I had cut my eyes at him. "Except that she had an affair with a man who had a wife and a small child, and I didn't and wouldn't. You know, except that."

Eric had inhaled slowly. "What I mean is that you are both intelligent and ambitious—good at your jobs. There were so many times when I was with Katrina that I would tell her how great you are. Once I was in it, I couldn't figure out a way to tell you without hurting you."

No, there had been no way to tell me and not hurt me. I had been through the hurting, the anger, and the betrayal. I had done a lot of healing. Maybe I was ready for growth because, in addition to wrinkling my nose at the strangeness of Eric's proposal, I was curious not only about that side of Eric but also about that side of the sexual tracks.

A few years earlier, before Will was born, Eric and I had embarked on a brief exploration with our next-door neighbors. They were a childless couple like us. On clear evenings, we relaxed in the spa on their back deck. They discouraged swimsuits, saying something about the detergent in them causing bubbles. Our evening respites involved talking about community politics and sipping wine.

One night, naked and flushed after the hot tub and alcohol, we had ended up on their living room carpet, talking in the dark. The husband and I moved closer to each other. The wife and Eric did the same. I suspected the husband had a little crush on me, and I was flattered. Eric used to tease me about it. He liked that the husband found me attractive.

It had been over a decade since I had kissed anyone other than Eric, and I wondered how it would feel. We exchanged a few gentle kisses on the lips, and he slowly caressed my breasts and belly. I felt a shiver at the novelty, although not much chemistry. I felt awkward but safe with Eric almost within reach. I assumed that Eric and the wife engaged in similar explorations, although I was not watching them, and I could see little in the shadows. No one got upset or stormed out. The encounter lasted less than twenty minutes. We said our good nights and got dressed.

On the half-block walk home, Eric asked, "What did you think?"

"I don't know." I paused to consider how I felt. "It was sort of flattering."

"Would you want to do that again?"

"Not especially. He's not my type. How about you? I didn't think she was your type."

Eric said, "It was kind of fun and a little exciting, but you're right. She's not my type. Plus, since you and I are trying to start a family, the timing doesn't seem good." Several months later, I was pregnant with Will. We had dropped any more experimenting until Eric's birthday request.

"Okay," I said. "It's your birthday. I guess I can try to keep an open mind, but no promises."

"Great to hear," Eric said. "Now, I want to suggest something additional."

Pushing it, aren't we, bud?

"There's another club less than an hour from The Lodge," he began. "Since we will be in the area for the weekend, how about we try The Lodge on Friday and The Ranch on Saturday? The Ranch is bigger, and Saturdays are supposedly the more popular nights."

There were two of these freaky places within spitting distance? And, come on, these club names sounded like a cowboy wannabe's wet dream of a sexy hoedown. Assaulting me behind my eyelids were unwelcome visions of a B-movie starring Ronald Reagan, riding bareback, wearing nothing but chaps, as he reached down from his trusty steed to pull up a tallow-haired cowgirl, sporting braids and dressed in a red calico thong and mid-calf, tasseled boots.

What the hell. In for a penny, in for a pound.

"Sure, we can try both. If I can't stand the Friday night club, we can skip the Saturday one, right, Eric?"

He smiled. "Fair enough."

Eric signed us up. We packed a bottle of my favorite Captain Jack's Spiced Rum because patrons brought their own booze. The club provided the setups. The Lodge was in a rural area, and finding it took us a while. There were no signs. I was mildly disappointed not to spy an arrow framed in flashing lights that announced, SEX PARTY THIS WAY! Nor was there even a tasteful marker depicting a log cabin emitting a cozy curl of chimney smoke and announcing THE LODGE, like an in-joke to those in the know.

We followed the directions provided via email, and after only one wrong turn, we pulled into a low-lit gravel lot. Eric parked and turned off the car. I looked over my shoulder at a nondescript door that was probably the entrance.

"How are you doing?" Eric asked.

"Okay," I breathed. "I don't know what to expect. Do you?"

"Not exactly, but from what I've read on the site, it's couples-only tonight, no single guys. I figure we just see how it goes. If something happens, cool. If not, then I'm here with my gal, and we can do what feels right. It's an adventure."

Inhaling deeply, I nodded. "Let's do this."

I was surprised that Eric's affair had not appreciably diminished my trust in him. For a while, I had tried to play the part I thought I was expected to play as the jealous, wronged, suspicious wife, but Eric's actions made that posture insincere. He offered me the password to his email account. I accepted. He answered every question I posed about where he was and what he was doing, including if he was looking at porn or blogs or chatting with female friends. I checked his emails and browsing history, but the frequency and energy I devoted to the tasks abated more each week.

I had known Eric to be an honest person who loved me and whom I could depend on and be my true self with for so many years that I found it hard to muster more than a spoonful of *I can't trust that cheating snake ever again.* In college, when Eric told his adored mother that he was in love with me and that we would decide how to raise any children and in what faith, even though different than hers, I knew that I was first in his life, as he was in mine. There was never a doubt that he respected my opinion and my intellect. He would tell friends and family that his grades improved after he started dating me. When I declined dates with him because I had to study, he studied with me.

Shortly after I relocated from Texas to Washington, DC, for law school, he followed, quickly finding a full-time job as well as an officer slot at a military reserve unit. I admired his competence and diligence. He beamed with pride at my every accomplishment, from law review and a coveted clerkship to my first jury trial, which he insisted on attending so he could "see me in action." I never doubted his love and commitment to me. At times, I wondered how I could have gotten so lucky. I would confide my apprehension to him: "It's so easy for us now. It makes me wonder when the bad times will come and how we will weather them." He would kiss me and tell me that whatever the future had in store, we would face it together.

Still, I chastised myself. Was I a traitor to feminism for taking him back and trusting in him? Trusting in us? Maybe. I didn't know. What I did know was how I felt. The energy required to live in a constant state of suspicion was exhausting. I chose to view Eric's proposal to attend a swingers club as a couple, and meet others as a couple, to be a show of his trust in me and his faith in us to move past the affair and on to something else.

I reasoned that it was no easy task to share what others saw as deviant behavior, even with, or perhaps especially with, someone you loved and respected. The club presented Eric with a means to explore his curiosity without lying. Maybe the desire for sexual variety, coupled with honesty, was the genesis of being married and swinging, back when our spouse-swapping fore-apes swung down from the trees and into the suburbs and handed us a bowl for car keys and condoms.

Part of me could not fathom that I was setting foot into a club with an address like State Road 49, where I might end up having sex with another man for the first time since college. How was this happening to me, the woman who had vowed a lifetime of monogamous love in front of family, friends, and the campus rent-a-rabbi?

* * *

We arrived at The Lodge early in the evening because new members were required to complete an orientation process. We each were handed a stack of forms. We read the club rules and acknowledged in ink that we knew not to touch anyone without permission, that clothes were required on the dance floor, and that an open door to a private room meant you could enter, but a closed door meant you could not. We confirmed that we were not law enforcement and promised that we would not take photographs. The receptionist gave us name stickers to show we were a couple. On my badge, Eric's name was printed below mine in parentheses. Our stickers were light blue, a color broadcasting that we were first-timers.

Fridays were couples-only nights. Saturdays were open to single men. Single women were always welcome because a single woman might hook up with a couple. Bisexual single women, I came to learn, were somewhat disparagingly called *unicorns* in reference to the hunt performed by some couples seeking a creature who would spark a fire in their marriage by desiring both the male and the female of the couple equally. Like a unicorn, they were so rare as to be mythical.

We patted our name stickers onto our chests and were ready to get the lay of the club. A smiling older woman greeted us warmly. She had white hair, and I guessed she was in her late sixties. She could have stepped out of a Betty Crocker ad if Betty Crocker had been a swinger. (Maybe she was. How do you know?) She and her husband were the owners.

"Hello! Welcome to The Lodge. Time for the nickel tour." She offered a brief backstory of the founding and operation of the club and, directing her comments primarily to me, assured me in grandmotherly fashion that the patrons were respectful and that I should never, ever do anything that made me uncomfortable.

"Honey, no means no. End of story." I nodded. I was not a kid. I had a kid. I knew how to take care of myself, but I appreciated her approach. I felt more at ease knowing the owners' philosophy.

She led us to a dinner buffet that reminded me of a summer camp dining hall. I learned that it was not uncommon at swinger clubs for dinner to be included, along with snacks such as pizza or wings at various times during the night. As the morning dawned, a light breakfast buffet might be offered. Meals and snacks were opportunities to meet new people or dine with people you already knew. Couples who knew each other might plan to meet at the club for dinner, dancing, and intimacy.

We met the bartender and handed him our bottle of rum. He affixed to it a one-inch square white sticker with a number written in black marker and told us to remember the number so when we wanted a drink, he would use our liquor. Next, we were shown the dance floor and the pool tables. We were told that there would be icebreaker activities on the dance floor, and after midnight, it was okay to dress in lingerie in the public areas if we so chose. I assumed Mama Crocker meant me. In the restroom, I saw baskets stocked with condoms, lube packets, deodorant, mouthwash, lotion, and hairspray.

I took Eric's hand as we followed Mrs. Crocker upstairs. She explained that the playrooms were first come, first served. If a door was closed, the room was in use. There were clean sheets on the beds and new sets in bins beside them. After use, it was courteous to remove the sheets. Most of the rooms had a double bed and a nightstand with condoms, lube, and towels. Some had two beds.

One room had a suspended, cushioned chair for sex play. Another room had what we figured out later was a spanking bench. It reminded me of a shortened pommel horse from my delusional grade school attempts to mimic Olympic gymnasts.

Most of the doors had windows. "Shade up means you're welcome to watch," our host explained. "Shade down means you're not."

A larger room held three double beds pushed together. Eric whispered, "For group sex." Mrs. Crocker said, "This door is always open. People can watch or participate."

We walked downstairs to a large room with a massage table and stored our backpack in a locker.

"Any questions for me, dears?" she asked. I had silently taken in all the tour stops.

I shook my head.

"No. I think we've got it, thanks," said Eric.

"Have a nice evening then." She smiled and went on her way, her brown loafers sliding along the carpet.

It was still early when our tour concluded. The club hadn't filled up yet.

"Shall we have some dinner?" Eric asked.

"Sure," I said. I felt like the new kid at school, absorbing everything and trying not to draw hasty conclusions, but alert for whatever might come. I wanted to stay open-minded to Eric's proposal.

The buffet consisted of a series of aluminum trays holding cooked meats, mashed potatoes topped with melting pats of butter, and soggy mixed vegetables that I guessed had been dumped from industrial-sized cans. Slices of peach pie and chocolate layer cake sat on small plastic plates in the muted shades of pale yellow and grayish blue found in city hospitals and middle schools.

Mystery meat was not the meal I had anticipated before an evening of sex with strangers, but this was all so new to me that I had no idea if it was typical. Besides, I was grateful for most meals I didn't have to prepare.

We carried our dinners to an empty table. "Is it what you expected?" I asked Eric.

"I guess?" he said. "What about you?"

"I think I expected it to be, I don't know, sleazier, flashier? More Playboy Mansion and less Motel 6," I said.

Eric laughed. "I know what you mean. You still game?"

"I am." I smiled and slid my hand toward his across the table, between our plastic plates. He placed his warm, strong hand on mine as naturally as he had been doing since college when he gazed at me in wonder as if he couldn't believe his luck.

After we finished eating, we wandered toward the bar. Lubrication seemed prudent. We nursed our drinks at the bar and engaged in small talk with other patrons. It felt like a teen party in a basement rec room where the lights were too bright and the music was too loud, awkward at first until the "fun" people showed up. I felt self-conscious, wondering if I was dressed appropriately. Too dressy? Too casual? Not slutty enough?

I had not been sure about the dress code because the website gave a lot of latitude. I had chosen a short swing dress, silver hoop earrings, and black cage heels that showed off my scarlet pedicure. Eric wore a tight-fitting, short-sleeved maroon shirt, black jeans, and black boots. It was a look I always found sexy on him.

I was more curious than nervous to see how the evening would play out. I wondered who showed up at a secluded swinger club. Married couples like us? May-December partners? Younger, older, Blacker, whiter? Highly educated or not as much? I was clueless as to how we would even start a conversation with a potential couple. I hoped Eric knew more about swinger mating habits.

Through it all, Eric remained upbeat. He was probably trying to preempt any mounting wariness or general negativity on my part. In our wedding photos, he appeared serious and intense, while I was smiling dreamily. When I asked about his demeanor, Eric said he was trying to keep me grounded, so I wouldn't break down during the ceremony. Maybe that was what he was doing at the club.

The place had the feel of a low-rent nightclub, but it was not without its charm. Eric and I played a round of pool. We participated in the icebreaker games on the dance floor, including passing an apple under our necks, which forced patrons to interact physically. We chatted with people at the bar. The talk was oddly typical.

"Hi, I'm Celeste, and this is my boyfriend, Mason. I see your blue tags. Is this your first time here?" Mason was wearing jeans and a plaid shirt with snaps. He was balding and carrying about fifty pounds extra. Celeste's bust was busting out of her low-cut nylon dress, and she was balancing impressively on strappy stilettos.

We shook hands all around. "Hi, Celeste, Mason. Yes, we're newbies. I'm Eric, and this is my wife, Natalie. Where are you guys from?"

We traded a few more pleasantries about the food and how often they came to the club.

"The crowd is a bit livelier at The Ranch. Have you been?" asked Mason.

"Not yet. Tomorrow," I said.

"Be sure to check out the hot tub," said Celeste. "It's huge!"

I could not discern their agenda, if any, from their body language, and I wasn't interested in pursuing anything physical with them. We made a polite exit to refresh our drinks.

Once we were safely at the bar, Eric asked, "What did you think?"

"He's not my type, but she was pretty enough," I said.

"Yeah, I could see he was not for you. I think she might have been into me."

"How does that work? I mean, if you like one half of the couple, and I don't like the other?" I asked.

"I guess it doesn't," said Eric. "Everyone has to be interested."

We scoped out couples at the bar and on the dance floor. Eric asked me if anyone caught my attention. "Not really. There aren't a lot of people here," I said. "Do you see anyone you'd like to talk to?"

"Not at the moment. How about we walk around?"

"Sure." I carried my drink as if it were an elixir that would cure my awkwardness.

We wandered, peeking into the rooms. Porn played on a few television screens, but that held no interest for me. I was not a watcher. Eric enjoyed a spectacle, so he liked the group rooms. Watching others, even from our vantage point outside the open-doored room, made me nervous. At midnight, many women changed into lingerie. The private rooms started filling up.

When it became clear that we would not be popping our swinger cherries with any other Lodgers, we found an empty room for ourselves. I did not drive all the way out to bumfuck not to get laid by someone, even if it was Eric rather than a steamy stranger.

"Door open or closed?" Eric asked.

"Door closed, but the shade can be open," I compromised.

The shade up meant we would have sex with the possibility of a stranger watching us. Being neither a voyeur nor an exhibitionist, that was a leap for me. At one point, I noticed a face in the window. I turned my head to block it out. It did not creep me out so much as distract me. When we were done, taking advantage of being as loud as we wanted, we were more than a bit pleased that we had broken the seal on this little adventure.

We didn't hook up with another couple at The Lodge, but we took the first step. I was growing more interested in what the next night would bring at the Saturday club: The Ranch.

* * *

The Ranch was bigger than The Lodge and had more private rooms. We dropped off our BYO booze, ate the standard fare buffet dinner, and stood at the edge of the dance floor, taking in the layout and the Saturday night vibe. The deejay was playing Katy Perry's "I Kissed a Girl." It was the first time I had heard the song, which I would later learn was a swinger club favorite.

I listened for a beat or two. "Fun song. Shall we dance?" I asked Eric.

"Following you," he said.

The Ranch started filling up. It was not long before a guy in his fifties, wearing jeans and a checkered shirt, danced close to me and started a conversation. "You're very pretty. I like the way you dance." I was flattered, but I wasn't attracted to him. We danced together, though, and that loosened me up. I spotted Eric chatting up a curvy, long-haired brunette, and he motioned me over. I was glad for an excuse to break free of my dance partner, which I politely did.

"Natalie, meet Alicia and her husband, Kenneth. This is their first time at the club, too."

I greeted everyone, and we made small talk. They seemed pleasant enough. I heard a song I liked and said, "Excuse me, guys. I am going to go dance."

Eric joined me, and Alicia and Kenneth followed. We all danced to an old pop song, the alcohol working on me as intended. Then we went our separate ways.

Eric made a point of saying, "Maybe we will see you later in the hot tub."

"Maybe so." Kenneth winked.

I found Kenneth attractive and engaging, and he was not afraid to express interest, which was helpful for me. I was awkward at flirting since, *hello*, I was married, and I did not flirt anymore, if I ever had. Kenneth was clean-shaven, wore his brown hair short (which was my preference), and had a generous smile. I could see that Eric was into Alicia. She was curvaceous and full-breasted. Her long, straight hair was almost black. Eric and I were in our early thirties. I guessed that they were a few years younger. The evening seemed promising.

True to Celeste's word, the hot tub was impressive—at least twenty feet long and roughly kidney-shaped. Eric and I decided to join the human stew of a dozen people.

"Alicia and Kenneth, at two o'clock," I said to Eric.

Eric nodded. "Do you want to join them?"

"Okay."

We dropped our towels near the edge of the pool. No one wore suits. Somehow, group nudity reduced the weirdness level, although it did not erase it, at least for me.

I slid in, letting the water settle at clavicle level. While I had body image issues like everyone, I realized that I was objectively in good shape for the mother of a preschooler, or so I was told. That said, we were not enjoying an evening dip with neighbors we had lived next to for years. We had just met these people. We didn't even know their last names. Nevertheless, we pressed on.

Socializing while nude took the guesswork and some first-timer anxiety out of that pre-sex quandary of *What do they look like under their clothes?* and *Will my lopsided boobs turn him off?* and *Is my cock big enough for her?* and, ultimately, *Will we be physically attracted to each other?*

We talked with Alicia and Kenneth about typical things—where we lived, our kids, and vacations. We also talked about some less typical things—how long we had been in open marriages and our extramarital experiences. Then came the negotiation.

Eric took me aside. "If you are interested, you should talk to Alicia. In the swinger game, it's less threatening for the women to make the decisions."

I nodded. I was interested.

Wait. How did Eric know so much about this dynamic? The internet, I assumed. I tried not to think too hard about what to say. *Keep it short and smile*, I thought as I approached her.

"Alicia, can I talk to you for a minute?"

"Okay," she said. I could not read her, but I swallowed my doubt and dove in.

"Eric and I would like to go upstairs with you. Are you guys interested in that?"

She said, "Let me talk to Kenneth." She didn't jump for joy, but she didn't reject the proposal either. I didn't know what to think. This was strange on so many levels.

I walked back to Eric.

"What did she say?" he asked.

"She's going to talk to Kenneth."

Eric did not have time to quiz me further because Alicia came back almost immediately. It was a go.

In swinging, according to Eric, my guide on this sexventure, there was *soft swap* and *full swap*. Alicia and Kenneth were a soft swap couple. That meant oral sex but no intercourse. Soft swap was a common compromise, especially for those new to swinging. I probably would have been cool with full swap because I found the distinction between soft and full swap to be adolescent, but it was my first time, so I followed their lead.

My relative nonchalance that this was going to happen—that we were going to have sex with two people we had met less than two hours before—both surprised and grounded me. Eric had been my only lover in the dozen years since college. I had expected to be a nervous wreck at the thought of having sex with a stranger, but I wasn't.

Our potential first swinger partners were a couple we might have met at a PTA meeting. They were nonthreatening, easy to talk to, and possibly also apprehensive at the prospect of getting physical with us.

The four of us found an unoccupied private room. We paired off and started making out with each other's spouses. There was just enough room to walk around the full-sized bed and end table. Since the space was less than a hundred square feet, we were all aware of what was going on with each other.

I could see Eric was keeping an eye on me and my new partner to make sure I was okay. I appreciated that. I discovered that I was comfortable having sex with someone else and with my husband doing the same, only inches from me. I had no trouble separating sex from love or another level of intimacy. I didn't feel threatened or jealous. Rather, I was glad Eric was having a good time. I knew Eric was a wonderful lover and communicator, so I expected Alicia would enjoy herself. My joy in Eric's joy with another partner, I later learned, was an emotion that polyamorists called *compersion*, and that many new polyamorists struggled to find it in the stew of jealousy that polyamory may stir.

While I did not stare at Eric and Alicia, I glanced over a few times. I heard Eric ask Alicia, "Is this better . . . or this?" I saw his head between her legs and, later, hers between his. From the other sounds I heard, they both were enjoying each other.

Kenneth and I gelled fine, too. We started with gentle kisses, working our way down each other's bodies with lips, mouths, and fingers and checking in with each other about what worked better or not as well. I saw Eric look my way and grin when he caught my eye as I pleasured Kenneth.

When everyone was finished, we lounged on the shared bed and talked.

"I am glad we met you guys and that we all had our first time together," I said.

"Agreed," said Alicia. "I was nervous about how this would go."

"You seemed to get into the groove," said Eric, smiling. "I am certainly a fan."

"You guys are a lot of fun," added Kenneth, gazing at me. I blushed, flattered to be the focus of his compliment.

While Alicia had loosened up since my proposal on the side of the hot tub, I got the sense she had come to the club with less enthusiasm than her husband. Call it intuition, or just my picking up on a vibe of reticence or caution because it mirrored what I had been feeling to some degree, this venture having been Eric's idea. I was to discover that it was not unusual for one spouse to be more into swinging than the other. The enthusiasm disparity was a constant balancing act in meshing with another couple.

Our swinger cherries popped, we said our goodbyes. It was two in the morning when we emerged from the small bedroom, and the club was almost deserted.

As was his way, Eric launched into the after-action review once he started the car.

"What did you like?"

"The naughty, sexy vibe; the excitement of someone new; seeing you enjoy someone else and pleasure someone else; being able to climax and bring someone else to climax; the flattery of being desired by someone else."

"What didn't you like?"

"The awkwardness of being in such close quarters; worrying if you and Alicia were having a good time; wondering if I could orgasm with a new partner and bring a new partner to climax."

I realized that I had not connected completely with Kenneth while we were all four on one bed. There was an artificiality to the encounter, as if we were on stage or being watched, because we were, even if the audience was a small, distracted one.

I added, "Kenneth was a fine lover and attractive enough, but he did not make me quiver like in a romance novel. I like having sex with you more. That realization is both disappointing and comforting if that makes sense."

"Yes, it makes sense," said Eric. "You rock my world, too, Natalie, but I won't deny it was an ego boost to know I could perform with someone else who was attracted to me and I to them." He paused. "Would you do it again?"

I considered. "Yes, I think so."

We were silent with our respective thoughts for a few moments.

Eric reached for my hand and brought it to his lips. The light in his eyes told me that he had had a very good birthday.

2.
The Lifestyle

After our night at The Ranch, Eric and I considered ourselves part-time swingers. While I was not a fan of that term, *lifestylers* was not much better. Over several years, we attended house parties, clubs, and sex-positive beach resorts. The experiences varied. Eric managed his expectations better than I did. He liked the atmosphere of the sexually open events where the women sported skimpy outfits. Even if we didn't connect enough with anyone to play with, Eric still enjoyed the view.

Play was another term I found incongruous. Swingers referred to sexual encounters as *play dates* and *playing* with others. It sounded like what children did in the sandbox, not what adults did in bed. That said, I didn't have a better word.

In our marriage, Eric was an extrovert, voyeur, risk-taker, kink appreciator, and happy to play in public. I was more of an introvert, not an exhibitionist, and risk-wary, with a preference for private play, whether kinky or vanilla. While Eric never met a stranger he could not charm, it took energy for me to engage in small talk. That made swinging a challenge for me because we met new people each time. While I didn't have moralistic qualms about swinging, I didn't get the charge out of it that Eric did. Doing what was seen as taboo solely because it was labeled as such was not a compelling reason for me to engage.

In swinging, one couple typically played in the same room with another couple. Eric and I being equally attracted to the partners in another couple was rare. I soon discovered that more often the woman was hot, engaging, and attractive, and the man was, well . . . not, at least not to me. This was frustrating to Eric because it meant a no-go, but he did not disagree that his options were usually better than mine. Eric appreciated a wide variety of women; I was attracted to lean, short-haired, relatively clean-shaven men who could carry on a conversation about something more than sports and porn.

During our six years or so as swingers when we were in our thirties, we met up with other couples sporadically. Many months could pass between encounters. It was a project to date other couples. Eric took charge of exploring the online sites, making the first cut of potential partners, and sending them messages. We were busy with work, family, and other social commitments. Having sex with men other than my husband was not my top priority. Eric's hierarchy of needs varied from mine.

I tended to go along with his suggestions for meetups or happy hours, often grudgingly because I doubted that I would find someone attractive after expending energy to socialize. I let Eric do the heavy lifting and did my part by being arm candy and trying not to roll my eyes or scowl when anyone was looking.

Before Eric's birthday present, I had been pretty *vanilla*, a catch-all label alternative communities used to distinguish themselves from the *normies* who pursued a more traditional, non-adventuresome lifestyle, such as monogamy. Before our swinger club initiations, the most dangerous thing I had done was pull Eric into an empty college classroom for quick sex in a plastic chair attached to an apostrophe-shaped desk and smear a wet streak on the chalkboard as my deviant calling card.

Nor had I tested my sexuality in college with other girls. I had not had a threesome, a foursome, or a moresome with people I had just met or whose names I never knew. I had not had sex in front of anyone but the person I was having sex with. I had never had sex with a hot stranger while my husband egged us on, or participated, or while guys I did not know watched me like I was a porn show, and I tried not to see them. I had never brought home a couple from a club to fool around in our basement. But, in time, I did all those things.

Those experiences made me someone other than the straight arrow, straight A, straight-haired, straight-and-narrow Natalie I had been all my life. I had a steamy secret side, but so what? I didn't know if that was what I wanted. Our swinging had not bruised any moral code or triggered jealousy, but for me, the novelty wore off quickly. *Okay, the sex with strangers box is checked, but what's in it for me . . . ?*

I was ready for something else, something that felt like more, even if at the time I didn't have a name for it.

3.

Swimming Upstream

Several years after our visits to The Lodge and The Ranch, we were living in an apartment while our house was being built. Absorbed in parenting, careers, and daily life, we had done very little swinging. I didn't miss the distraction as much as Eric did.

Each weekday morning for six months, I drove from our rental apartment to our son's elementary school, drove back to the rental, parked the car, and caught a bus to the train to my office. Too often, my day started with me impatient with ten-year-old Will to get ready for school and ended with me rushing to handle meal prep and laundry. I was beat. While Eric impressively dealt with the home-building logistics, becoming an expert on the local building code and architectural software, the large-scale project was demanding and stressful.

Our sex life suffered, and it was taking a toll on Eric, so when Eric told me that a band he liked was touring the East Coast, performing three concerts in three cities in as many days, and he wanted to go, I listened.

"I've mapped it out," he said, "and I can drive to each one. I'm pretty sure I can find a friend to go with me for company and to share the driving and expenses."

"I know you could use the break. Go ahead and have fun. I'll stay with Will."

When Eric told me who had responded with interest to his offer to see the shows and share hotel room costs, my enthusiastic support for the road trip waned.

Eric knew Lorraine from the goth and electronic music scene, and she was a fan of the touring band. She was a sometime deejay with a reputation for being difficult. Eric considered Lorraine fun and adventuresome, two adjectives he would not have used to describe me then. Lorraine had been married a couple of years to a guy who rarely accompanied her on the goth and '80s club outings where I would run into her, so I knew little about him. I judged Lorraine as flighty and irresponsible. She had trouble keeping a job, and even Eric admitted she was no Rhodes Scholar. She had made flashcards to study for her driving test and still failed it twice. I guessed she was in her mid to late thirties, half a dozen years younger than me.

I had no concrete reason not to trust Eric and Lorraine on the trip. Since the affair with Katrina, there had been no indiscretions that I was aware of. Our foray into swinging had been a consensual co-adventure.

Still, I said to Eric, "Please don't sleep with her."

"We are just going to see a few shows."

"I know the travel itinerary, Eric. I am asking you not to sleep with her."

He sighed. "That was eight years ago, Natalie."

I wanted to trust him and to trust that our life and our relationship were on track. I also wanted him to know that I was not blind to the fact that things at home were stressful, and that we were still at risk. His infidelity with Katrina had torn a corner of my heart, and I could feel the stitches straining. When he called from the car to say he and Lorraine were on their way to the first concert, and I heard their laughter, I was glad he was happy. I wanted him to be happy. But I was wary.

After the road trip, our life continued as it had. Eric and I still shared a computer. He still left windows open, which slowed down our early 2000s processor when I used it. As I was closing an email window, I saw a message about him meeting Lorraine for lunch. My heart raced. *Jesus Fucking Christ. Not again.* I understood what it meant to feel your blood boil. I told myself to calm down. He wouldn't be careless enough to make the same mistake twice. Eric was smarter than that.

Eric was in the other room. Will was not in bed yet. I could wait.

Later that evening, I asked Eric to sit down.

"Eric, are you sleeping with Lorraine?"

"What? No. Why would you ask that?"

I said, "I saw an email you left open talking about meeting her for lunch. This is how I found out about Katrina, so please don't tell me I'm paranoid."

"Lorraine is trying to get back into deejaying, and she asked for my advice," he said. "She's burned some bridges in the local goth scene because she can be a bit of a diva. I said I would talk to her about some ideas. She doesn't drive, so I offered to come to her. I feel sorry for her."

"Just advice to a friend," I said.

"Yes," he said.

"That's very generous of you," I said.

I did not raise the matter again. We were busy with the house building. Once the spring weather became drier, the foundation was laid, and construction began in earnest. Then, in early summer, I suffered an injury.

Two months after Eric's road trip with Lorraine, I broke my right arm, sliding into second base during a summer weekend game with my coed softball team. A ball thrown to the shortstop pounded me, rather than his glove, with such force that it left the imprint of the ball's seam on my forearm. Eric slogged through awful traffic to rescue me from the dugout. I was sweaty, dirty, and whimpering in self-piteous pain.

From the immediate vicinity of the ball field, Eric scavenged a two-by-four almost a yard long, secured it under my arm with an abandoned plastic grocery bag, and fashioned a brace to alleviate the pain while he drove me to the emergency room. I had six casts of varying colors in as many months. The final two were as black as my mood.

I was so right-hand dominant that I had to come up with creative ways to function. At work, I started using voice recognition software to draft briefs. It was cumbersome and slow, but I could not type on a keyboard. Forget grasping a pen. I had to sign documents left-handed. My signature was a lopsided, squiggly, hesitant mess as if I were a six-year-old trying to forge my mother's signature. Maybe I had missed my calling as a physician.

I taught myself to operate a doorknob with my left hand, thinking hard about which way to turn it. For the first few weeks, I did not feel safe driving with Will in the car. Cooking for my family was also a challenge because I couldn't chop anything.

The apartment we rented over a restaurant had two small bedrooms and a bathroom downstairs that we were not using. Eric suggested that while my arm was healing, we offer that space for someone to live in and help with cooking, errands, driving, and housework. Eric wrote an ad and interviewed applicants, and we agreed on a lovely young woman in her late twenties who was temporarily in the area to see family. The barter arrangement with Helen was a lifesaver.

Soon after I broke my arm, Eric and I drove Will to a two-week summer camp. We planned to take an extra day for ourselves on the way back at a bed and breakfast Eric had found. He loved castles, and the tiny house had a turret. We arrived late and slept in, deliciously reconnecting our bodies, fitting into the grooves we had worn into each other over the decades. I luxuriated in the realization that we had no obligation for the day before driving home. We could wander the town or go on an adventure.

After breakfast, we sat in a gazebo, shaded from the late morning sun. I felt more peaceful than I had in weeks, despite the periodic throb of my broken arm.

"I need to tell you something, Natalie."

I looked across the octagonal divide at Eric. His palms cupped his chin as he leaned his elbows on his knees. I braced myself as if for a physical blow.

Eric told me that he had slept with Lorraine on the road trip. He had not planned it. They were sharing a hotel room because she could not afford her own. She had made the first move, and he had not objected.

The midday rendezvous I saw in the email was for sex while her husband was at work. Eric thought her husband had come home at lunch one day and heard them, so their affair was likely over. Eric told me he had felt disconnected from me and undesired, as if he were one more chore on my list of things to do. With Lorraine, he felt desired.

Out came his confession, like the high tide pounding the shore. I absorbed the impact like body blows, barely flinching.

"When I asked you if you were sleeping with her, you lied to my face? You let me think I was paranoid."

"Yes, I lied," he said. "It wasn't the right time to have this discussion. I knew we would be alone on this trip soon, and Will would be at camp. I didn't know how it would go, if you would kick me out. I had to be ready for that."

"You were planning to talk to me today, after the great sex we just had?"

"I thought it might be the last sex we ever had. It was great," Eric said, holding my gaze. "Having sex with you is my favorite thing in the world. It always has been."

I sat in silence. My shoulders sagged. I felt the energy drain from me and form a dark puddle at my feet.

I was flattered that he enjoyed our sex life so much, but I felt played, and not for the first time. He had anticipated it might be our last time, although only he knew that. Even after agreeing, in an honest and consensual way, to open up our marriage to swinging, this had happened a-fucking-gain. Consensual non-monogamy, at least our swinging version, did not include his sleeping with someone and hiding it from me.

Admittedly, it had been eight years since the affair with Katrina, but I couldn't deny he was a repeat offender. What was it about me that caused him to cheat? I was hard to get along with. I was impatient and judgmental. And now, I was partially helpless with a broken arm. At least this time, I had a job.

"Do you want me to move out?" he asked.

"No," I said. "What do you want?"

"I want to stay," he said, "if you'll have me."

I was filled with more loathing for myself than for him. I blamed Lorraine, of course. *Whore*, *slut*, *moron*, *liar*, *cheat*, and *harlot* were some of the more charitable monikers I assigned her. I found it hard to blame Eric because if I had, I would not have been unable to justify loving him, valuing him, and wanting to keep our family together. I sensed that Eric, as a divorced father, might very well be an absent one. I didn't want that for Will. I needed to protect my family unit.

I silently vowed that I would be better. I would be a better wife, a better person. I would prioritize time with Eric. I would not kick Eric out, and I would not leave him. I would fix it. I would fix me. The thought of breaking up my family made my stomach churn. It made me feel like a failure. I hated myself for not being stronger, but my life was tied up with Eric. We were partners in so many ways. His affair with Lorraine had not changed that. It had only confirmed how far he would go to feel sufficiently desired, if not by me, then by someone else.

We wandered the grounds of the small property. He talked. I listened. We both shed some tears. After a few hours of examining our relationship and our lives, we started the drive home. Eric would stop seeing Lorraine. We would try to find more space for us amid the daily grind.

I remember stopping for dinner, my throbbing arm propped up on the table to alleviate some pain, and thinking that no one in the restaurant knew how I had spent my day. They did not know that I was swallowing guilt, pain, and shame with my dinner. Eric was soft-spoken and kind to me across the table, which made me feel even worse, as if he was the better person, and I was the intolerant, selfish, demanding shrew even though he was the one who had lied and cheated on me.

There we sat, two people flawed and hurting, eating fish on a weekend in June, each deep inside our heads contemplating what would happen next. We had two weeks while Will was at camp to figure that out.

Over those weeks, I thought and rethought my decision to stay with Eric. After a massive amount of reflection, beating myself up, and communicating with Eric, by which I mean crying, cursing, sleeping apart, sleeping together, and considering if I would be better off shed of him, we stayed together and moved on. Eric broke up with Lorraine. Lorraine's husband kicked her out. Will came home from camp. I left the laundry unfolded, making deliberate efforts to spend time, particularly sex time, with Eric and communicate that I desired him.

There was collateral damage. In an email, Lorraine called me a doormat for taking Eric back. That smarted. Eric told her she had no right to judge our more than twenty-year relationship and that he would not tolerate the woman he loved being called that. Lorraine took it back, saying she was envious that our relationship was stronger than hers and her husband's.

I tried to let it go, but the word *doormat* haunted me. Was I? I swallowed the insult and tried not to choke on self-pity. *No*, I told myself. *I am stronger than that. My marriage is stronger than that. Screw you, Lorraine. You lost, not me.*

Six months later, in January 2009, we moved into our new house. I watched a historic presidential inauguration on television as I unpacked boxes. We settled into our routine. Will could walk to school again. My commute to work was shorter by half. Eric did not have the house project to contend with.

Helen moved with us from the apartment to the house to continue helping us while she waitressed part-time. She stayed with us for two years. We all breathed easier.

4.
Say What?

Less than a year after his affair with Lorraine, Eric was sitting in an armchair reading, and I was at the shared computer planning a trip for the family over Will's winter break. Since the move, swinging had not been on my radar much. Eric was on some lifestyle sites, and we had attended a few swinger house parties, but Will's sports, school, and PTA, as well as getting settled in the house, took up most of our time.

Eric said, "Natalie, you know how we talked about opening up our relationship and seeing other people separately, rather than swinging? Well, I know who I'd like to see."

Say what? I thought. *I don't remember those discussions. Maybe I wasn't listening or hoping it was a phase that would pass, but okay, I'll play along.*

"Oh?" I asked. "Who?"

Eric said, "Well, there's an obvious choice."

"There is?" I asked.

"Lorraine," he said.

Silence.

More silence.

"What?" I asked.

Eric said, "We get along. We have fun. I enjoy her company. We like a lot of the same things."

Incredulous silence.

I don't recall the exact discussion. It is quite possible that I said something like, "Are you fucking kidding me?" That sounds like how I would have responded, at least at first. Or maybe I swallowed hard, thought about it, and realized that it made some sense. Likely, I did both.

As I recall, I exercised extreme restraint in not throwing something as I listened and chewed on my response. I concluded that it took considerable courage, or chutzpah, depending on your perspective, for Eric to tell the mother of his child, his chosen life mate, and the woman he cheated on more than once that he wanted to date someone else, and that someone else was the slut he had had an affair with.

I did not mouth off what was in my head because I was a pragmatist. The end of Eric's affair had not ended his needs, nor transformed me into Eric's ideal partner. Despite my efforts, I still struggled with impatience and stress levels. Those criticisms by Eric were legitimate. I had started seeing a therapist to help me devise strategies to manage anger, parent more patiently, and deal with life stresses in less caustic ways, without rocketing from mild-mannered to Medusa in a minute.

"I guess if you want to date Lorraine, you can, but I am not interested in dating anyone," I said.

I could not fathom dating when I had so much on my plate. I barely had the time or inclination to sleep with my husband, much less anyone else. My libido seemed so suppressed that I asked my physician about it. She joked that if she had a nickel for every woman with my complaint, she would be a millionaire, but there was no little blue pill for women. I was not laughing. The sum of her uninspired medical advice was that I was stressed, like millions of working mothers, and I should set aside a weekly date night with my husband.

"If I agreed to you dating Lorraine, how would it work?" I asked.

Eric told me that he had been reading about *polyamory*, a relationship dynamic where we could pursue separate relationships as individuals instead of as a couple dating a couple. We would be open and honest about who we dated and when. Informed consent by all participants and intentional communication were mandatory. There was no lying or cheating.

"If you are up for it, we can try it," Eric said. "If it isn't working, we can stop."

Eric gave me some non-monogamy books—from a small collection I didn't know he had—to help me get my head around the concept and how it might work for us. *The Ethical Slut* by Dossie Easton and Janet Hardy was a primer, first published in 1997, which used the term polyamory—*poly* for short. The term was credited as being coined in 1990 by Morning Glory Ravenheart Zell, a pagan priestess. *Polyamory* took its roots from Latin and Greek to mean "many loves." Eric also offered me Anthony Ravenscroft's 2004 treatise, *Polyamory.* I read some excerpts and skimmed for highlights, but I was not jazzed to add reading assignments to my list of responsibilities. I preferred talking with Eric to figure out what we needed to give polyamory a go. The idea that it was a relationship construct that could be tailored to individual circumstances sounded good to me. We could make our own rules.

The literature told me that it was not uncommon for polyamory to be discussed in the aftermath of an affair when a partner in a monogamous relationship who still loved their spouse wanted to open up the marriage without losing the primary relationship, but did not know how to do it in an honest way.

If I had learned anything from Eric's affairs and our sporadic foray into the swinger lifestyle, it was that Eric could and maybe even needed to have more than one love in his life. He seemed to be able to care for me and someone else simultaneously, fulfilling different needs and desires with different people. I was struck by how he seemed to genuinely feel not less love for me when he explored other relationships, but more. The concept of many simultaneous loves was so foreign to me that acknowledging its value and applicability to the real world, and in particular to my world and our marriage, was, shall we say, a process.

My first year of polyamory was one of the worst years of my life, even as I struggled to do my best—as we did *our* best—in wildly unfamiliar territory.

I had always found structure and schedules comforting, hence my chosen profession. Polyamory threw me. My control over my relationship, and my life, seemed to be wobbling on an unstable foundation. I felt as if Eric had kicked out one of the four legs under the dining room table and challenged me not just to keep it upright, but also to hold a steaming dinner for the family without scalding anyone, like a carnival clown.

I had no one to talk to about polyamory except Eric, and I felt alone. But, hell, I was a problem-solving, self-sufficient, pragmatic, twenty-first-century gal. I could figure this out. Right?

I would later conclude that if anyone was ever born polyamorous, that person was Eric. We just had not known there was a term for it. You might say, *ahem, there is a term for it, you weak-willed simp. Lying, cheating bastard is one that comes to mind.* As if I had not thought that already.

I tried all kinds of techniques to come to terms with the new dynamic. This foray into polyamory was different than swinging because I was not an active part of it. Eric would be dating and sleeping with another woman, in addition to me, but not *with* me. I would have no idea what was going on between my husband and his lover except what he told me. I was wracked with self-doubt.

And the feminist in me would not shut the fuck up. I would have dialogues out loud, but in a conversational, not too obvious tone, as I walked to the train station on my way to work, often with tears streaming down my face. Thank goodness for Bluetooth. Most people assumed—I hoped?—that I was on the phone, rather than talking to myself like a street person off her meds.

Voice in my head: *Have you no self-respect? Weren't you raised to be a strong, self-assured, self-sufficient woman who doesn't need a man?*

Me: *Yes* (I nodded), *I was.*

Voice: *How can you condone this? This arrangement means one thing. He is tired of you. You are not enough. Screw that and screw him. If he wants to sleep with other women, let him. Divorce his ass. It's the only self-respecting response to his proposal.*

Me: *But I love him. And he loves me. Oh my god, I can't believe I just said that. I sound like some abused wife with a black eye who thinks she deserves a beating. I hate my pathetic self. At least I think he does. I mean, he's being honest and having this conversation with me. I could say no to this, but I see that he needs it, and what harm is it to me, really?*

Voice: *Ha! This is love? "I love you, honey, but I want to sleep with other women—younger women—who I find more fun or more attractive or more something." How is that love? That is manipulation of your emotions. That is an "I dare you to say no and see what happens to your world."*

Me: *Do you think I am blind? I am not stupid. Don't ever call me stupid. I see all that, but I don't want a divorce. Just because this arrangement is unconventional doesn't mean it's wrong, or wrong for us. Maybe it's a growth experience, or maybe I am just a sniveling coward afraid to admit that my life is crumbling around me.*

Voice: *Well, let's not get all drama queen. Your life is not crumbling. Your husband is. Ditch him and move on.*

Me: *It's not that easy, and I don't want to. Why are you making me feel bad for giving this a try, for believing him when he says he loves me and acts like he does as well?* (Deep inhale, slow exhale.) *I am trying this. I want to trust myself and my husband and see where it takes me.*

My internal narrative was an unproductive maze. What helped me move out of its tracks was communicating with real people who knew me and understood polyamory. In addition to Eric, I discovered a few trusted friends who were patient and considerate enough to let me voice my fears and frustrations and to listen with empathy and offer rational perspective. They saved my life, or at least my sanity.

How did the girl in the princess-sleeved wedding dress, wearing her grandmother's pearls and vowing love and fidelity until death parted her from her beloved, become a joyfully polyamorous woman with lovers and boyfriends and a universe of romantic and non-romantic connections outside her marriage?

Stay tuned.

5.
Bad Penny

Lorraine was my first *metamour*, a word I had never heard before I agreed to try a polyamorous marriage and read the poly literature. A metamour is the other lover of your lover. They are your husband's girlfriend, your boyfriend's wife, your girlfriend's other girlfriend.

So there was a word for that. Great, but now what? I had a freighter's worth of questions. What was my relationship with this metamour person? What were my expectations, their expectations, my husband's or my lover's expectations? Did we all have to be best buddies, friendly acquaintances, confidantes, lovers, never meet each other, or just minimally tolerate each other?

It turned out that the answer to those questions was "it depends."

After warily agreeing to try this polyamory experiment, I discussed with Eric what our rules and expectations would be. When I look back at all the rules I needed, the current me shakes her head, but at the time, we agreed that rules were required. Eric acknowledged that his behavior had damaged the trust in our relationship. Eric was not one to lie, except, it turned out, about screwing other women. Before his cheating, it had been a given that we were upfront and honest with each other. I had found, oddly, that the affair with Katrina nearly a decade before had not made me a paranoid wife. We had dealt with what I viewed as an episode, not a permanent character flaw. Was I wrong?

If I had doubted Eric's love and long-term commitment to me, his dating Lorraine could not have gotten out of the starting gate. Eric was an open line of communication. He listened to me complain and vent about Lorraine. *I don't trust her. She wants you for herself and is just biding her time until you leave me. She texts you too much. She wants too much. I don't like her.*

He listened to my fears, both rational and irrational, and endured my sometimes selfish rules. *She can't be in our house. She can't ride on the back of the motorcycle. That's "our" thing. You can see her only twice a month.*

I kept copious mental notes of the number of dates they had, and if he exceeded the agreed allotment, I called him on it, and he canceled the date.

When Eric thought a rule was unreasonable, all he did was ask me to reconsider; many times I did, but sometimes I did not.

I needed rules to feel that the world I knew was not slipping out from under me. Rules were common in polyamory. The new relationship paradigm could not have functioned for us without them. Having rules was a necessary part of evolving to not having them.

Determining our rules involved discussing what we wanted and trying to accommodate our desires. We also addressed what Lorraine wanted from our letter V-shaped relationship structure. A *hinge* is the partner at the point or hinge of a three-person poly relationship. In our case, I was one *arm* of the V. Lorraine, my metamour, was the other. Eric was the *hinge.*

As our hinge, Eric communicated to me what Lorraine wanted. Some polyamorists have three-way conversations or meetings, but that was not us, at least at that early stage. I disliked Lorraine, so I kept our interactions minimal. Eric was responsive to Lorraine's needs as well as to mine and communicated well as our hinge. And so the negotiations commenced.

From Eric, Lorraine wanted regular dates, as often as possible, regular contact by email, text or phone, affection, consideration, and access. She wanted a friend, a lover, and ultimately, I concluded, she wanted Eric to herself. Eric disagreed with my assessment of Lorraine's motives, despite corroboration by mutual friends. Debating the issue proved frustrating and fruitless. I eventually stopped mentioning it.

From Lorraine, Eric wanted regular dates, sex, adventures, escape from the everyday, and the ability to easily extract himself.

From me, Eric wanted consideration. Compersion would have been nice, but my tolerance and civility were the bare minimum.

It was also important to Eric that the three of us met periodically and interacted courteously. He liked us to go out together to a club or restaurant to give a public face to our arrangement, so that it was clear that his dating Lorraine was not a dirty secret, that I was on board with the relationship, and that he was not a cheat.

For my part, I wanted advance knowledge of their dates, a defined number of dates per month, complete honesty, the right of first refusal for scheduling, their discretion and consideration, and as little contact as possible from Lorraine when Eric was with me during family hours. I did not want her in my home, and I preferred minimal communication between her and me. They could not take trips, and I had veto power, or so I thought, over a proposed outing and over the relationship with Lorraine or anyone else.

Eric was the one who mentioned *veto power*. My opinion in retrospect is that veto power is a construct that gives a sense of security to polyamory newcomers. It meant that I could prohibit an action or relationship, and he would acquiesce. As in, *Eric, I am vetoing you dating Shannon. She is a notorious conflict magnet and drama queen. I don't trust her.*

Neither Eric nor I exercised veto over a partner or potential partner in all our years of polyamory. When one of us expressed enough discomfort with, or excitement for, a new partner or activity, the other listened and tried to be considerate of their needs. Eric told me that he viewed veto power as a failsafe escape mechanism, to be applied if either of us could not see the irrevocable damage a relationship was causing to one of us or to our marriage.

I viewed rules as different from vetoes because rules were preestablished. Then again, a veto could become a rule. This came up when Eric wanted to take Lorraine on the motorcycle we had recently purchased. Holding on to Eric and feeling the bike under us on a clear day was something I treasured. I liked how Eric would look over his shoulder at me and smile or squeeze my leg with his leather-gloved hand. It was romantic, and the opportunities for us to ride were limited.

So I said no. I did not want her on our bike. Eric thought I was being inconsiderate and petty (I was) and asked me to reconsider. I thought about it and told him I didn't want Lorraine to ride with him because it was something I wanted to keep for us. What I did not say was that because I did not like Lorraine, I did not want her to enjoy the bike with him. That was really petty. Eric honored my request, and thus it became a rule that Lorraine was not allowed on the bike.

Rules like that were later scrubbed completely, but during the Lorraine era, I needed them. I needed to know that my wants and needs were heard, considered, and valued. At the crux, what I needed after Eric's cheating was to feel control in my relationship. Eric understood this and put up with a lot of what I came to think in hindsight was selfish and mean.

The rule that mattered most, and still does, was that we communicate. Eric and I spent countless hours sitting on our marital bed hashing and rehashing our relationship and his relationship with Lorraine. He listened to my fears and worries and kissed away tears with reassurances of his love for me and commitment to our life together.

"She is younger and more fun," I whined. "You would rather be with her."

"Natalie," he sighed, "I come home to you, to our bed, every time because that is what I want. I want you. I don't want to be with Lorraine all the time, just sometimes. I treasure our life together. I am grateful for the gift of polyamory that you give to me. I know how lucky I am."

Eric regularly checked in with Lorraine to take the temperature of their relationship, asking if she had any issues to discuss. Eric told me that he would pointedly remind Lorraine of the limits of their relationship. Namely, he loved me, he was not leaving me, and she and I being civil to one another was a necessity to the continuation of their relationship.

He told me that Lorraine would smile and nod and assure him that all was good except to ask if they could have a bit more time together, or plan an out-of-town trip, or something similarly negotiable. She would also tell Eric that she was not seeing anyone other than him because that was the way she wanted it and that seeing him twice a month was plenty. Lorraine told Eric that she liked having the space after her marriage had ended badly. She insisted she was not looking for a monogamous relationship and liked being on her own.

"Have you considered that maybe she is telling you what you want to hear?" I asked.

"No," Eric said. "Why would she lie?"

"To keep you, of course," I said. "Don't you see that she knows if she doesn't say that you will end the relationship?"

"Natalie, I have no reason to disbelieve her. I'm the one who is with her. I'm the one who sees how earnest she is. Don't you think you're being paranoid?"

"Me, paranoid? I wasn't the one who was sneaking behind my husband's back in his own home, screwing someone else's husband, now was I?" I huffed.

"Natalie . . ."

"Eric," I barreled on. "She told Trisha that she wanted you for herself, that she is just waiting for us to break up, that she had hoped that when her husband left her, I would toss you out too, right into her arms."

"You and I have had this conversation," Eric sighed. "All I can do is talk to her and take her at her word and observe her actions. She has done nothing to make me doubt that she is satisfied with the relationship as it is, other than wanting a little more time, which I told her I cannot give her. What more do you want me to do?"

Kick her to the curb like the trash she is, I thought but did not say. I did not want to be the reason for a breakup. There would always be a wedge between us if I were. He would eventually see her for who she was, or he wouldn't.

"Do you want me to break up with her?' Eric asked, as if on cue.

"No. I am not your mother. I am not going to tell you what to do, but I see things from a different perspective than you," I said.

As in, *Dude. Listen, I am not sleeping with her, so I am not blinded by lust. Snap out of it!*

I saw that Lorraine's actions were not necessarily congruent with her words. While she told Eric that she was happy with the status quo, she still asked for more time with him. I saw her calling and texting Eric often, and when he did not respond immediately, she got antsy. She bugged me to mediate, assist, and remind him of their scheduled dates. *What was I, his secretary?*

On more than one occasion, Lorraine contacted me, as if I were the impediment to Eric contacting her. Sometimes she would message me, "Eric is not responding to my texts, and I need to talk to him. Will you get him to call me?"

I was often aware she was contacting him because I could see the message alerts on his phone on the nightstand, or charger, or wherever he left his phone because he was not tethered to it. I would say, "Hey, Eric, Lorraine called you."

"I know," he would say.

When, one weekend, Lorraine convinced a mutual friend to call Eric and beg him to call Lorraine because he had not responded to her repeated calls and texts, even though there was no crisis, her intrusion and gall got on my last nerve. I was still learning that there are times when your partner's choice of a poly partner will not be your choice. It can boggle the mind.

"Eric, to me, Lorraine seems ditzy and irresponsible, which are not traits you value. You have told me that she is not too bright. She can't seem to hold a job, and many people we know have witnessed her gossiping and outbursts. It might help me get on board with your relationship and be more supportive if you could help me understand what (the hell!) you see in her."

Eric explained in words even a snippy, cheated-on wife could understand. "She's fun and easy to talk to. We like the same music and movies. She is up for anything, including stuff I know you're not, like sex clubs. Lorraine is grateful for the time we have together, whether that's fast food and a film or sushi and a hotel room. I don't see her as demanding. What you see as annoying or intrusive behavior, I see as manageable relationship noise."

He continued, "I know she may not be the brightest bulb, but that's not her fault. Her life has been a different road from yours. I don't need to date a rocket scientist. I already live with a competent, highly functioning woman. When I drop her off after a date, both of us are content and relaxed. I am grateful for my time with her and happy to come home to you."

Hearing Eric's perspective helped me understand. "Thank you for explaining. I suppose I could be more supportive. But please tell her I'm not your social secretary," I said, smirking.

I both appreciated and lamented that Lorraine was up for anything. On the one hand, that she was psyched to go to a clothing-optional kink camp where some people dressed like animals, some like babies, and many sought beatings that let them show off bruises that spread over their asses, backs and thighs saved me from exploring kink and *BDSM*—an acronym for Bondage and Discipline,

Domination and Submission, Sadism and Masochism—when I was not ready for it. *Kink* is unconventional erotic behavior that includes BDSM, exhibitionism, voyeurism, and fetishes. I heard the terms kink and BDSM used interchangeably, although BDSM is a type of kink. Those I knew who were into BDSM referred to themselves by the umbrella term *kinksters*.

On the other hand, Lorraine's willingness to be good and game for kinky activities highlighted, in my mind, that I was lacking. I was not fun enough, chill enough. I was too uptight, too straight. Nevertheless, my relief at not having to participate or feel guilty for saying no to those experiences outweighed my chagrin because I sincerely did not want to stand in the way of Eric living his fullest life. I was happier to step aside so he could take Lorraine to a metal concert or burlesque show. It was far better for her to bounce along with him to an event than for me to trudge after him and both our experiences be subpar.

About a year into his dating relationship with Lorraine, Eric and I were at a weeknight music recital to see Will perform with his elementary school orchestra. Lorraine had been calling Eric incessantly all evening. I was irritated at her intruding on a family event. From the snippets of conversation I overheard, Lorraine was hysterical and accusatory about something that happened on their recent date and was demanding he apologize for his wrongs. Eric tried to reason with her and finally said, "Fine, if you want to break up because of some perceived slight, then we are done."

Lorraine did not stay silent long. After a day or two, she kept turning up like a bad penny. She alternated between apologizing and begging him to come back and accusing him of using her and never genuinely caring for her. The push and pull between them went on for weeks. I could not fathom why he kept taking her calls and being polite but distant.

I wanted to shout, *Why don't you tell her to get lost already? Here, give me the phone. It will be my pleasure to do it for you. No charge.*

My initial elation at having her out of our lives smacked into the thundercloud of Eric's sullenness. I thought being rid of the Lorraine irritant would be good for our relationship. We would have time for us without her calls and messages and general presence. Who needed that pain in the ass? Not me for sure, and now Eric would see that she was more trouble than she was worth.

But Eric missed Lorraine. He forgave her for her impetuous demands, but he was not ready to get back together despite the tangible hole in his life without her. They had been seeing each other on the sly and then with my knowledge for two years by then.

The breakup with Lorraine did not make my life easier, nor bring Eric and me closer. Her absence highlighted that he, and maybe we, needed her, or needed *a* her. Our relationship of more than twenty years was in an ebb, not a flow. I could not put my finger on it, but the marital atmosphere was tense. Eric would leave for his first overseas military deployment in a few months. I found myself wishing he would go already to give us space. I sensed he felt the same.

Finally, after weeks of Eric's moodiness and the depressive effect on our relationship, I threw up my hands.

"You want to see her? Fine, go," I said. "That would be better than watching you mope around here wanting to." I said it partly in exasperation and partly in sympathy. While I did not want her back in our lives with her attendant drama that had oozed over me like slime, I could see that Eric missed her. I supposed I held out some hope he would decide not to see her, thereby validating my negative assessment of the content of her character and my positive, albeit wavering, assessment of the content of his.

He went to her. They had sex. Maybe he got closure. I didn't ask for details. I wouldn't have been surprised if they maintained occasional contact, but I found no evidence of it during my increasingly less frequent inspections of his phone.

The Lorraine episode demonstrated that there was no way a polyamory novice like me could have gotten my head and heart fully around accepting as my metamour the woman who cheated on her husband with my husband. After the humiliation I felt at their affair, my button had not only been pushed but permanently compressed. What had been born in the mire took stronger stuff than I was made of to pull it up to where civility lived.

I was not that evolved. I was angry and irritated, and I stayed that way for a long, long time. Even as I tried my damnedest to get on board, the year Eric dated Lorraine, with my knowledge and mostly informed consent, was awful. There were days I wanted unspeakably horrific things to happen to my husband's lover that involved, by way of example, an incurable flesh-eating disease. The intensity of my animosity toward another human scared me.

When I said that how a metamour relationship develops "depends," I meant it depends on circumstance and the individuals involved. Much as friendships, marriages, business associations, and familial relationships are dependent on the parties' expectations, agreements, and personalities, so too are metamour relations. Relationships are made up of people, and we decide which people we have to get along with, at least minimally, including in-laws, bosses, clients, and metamours, and which ones we can choose to walk away from.

However, despite what I thought my metamour was doing, feeling, or plotting, it was inexcusable for me to be unkind or to scheme to undermine her. I am not proud that I sent Lorraine emails feigning comradery and sympathy, all the while seething with contempt. When I suspected she and Eric had violated our rules by going to a neighborhood motel without my knowledge while I was out of town for work, I tricked her into admitting it by falsely telling her a friend of mine had seen our car in the motel parking lot.

My poly journey would come to include many different metamours. I learned and grew from those relationships. Lorraine was my first and not my best.

After Eric and Lorraine broke up, Lorraine was in a long-term monogamous relationship with someone who seemed to understand her and treat her well. Eric was happy she had found someone to love and care for her. His compersion was genuine. When I saw Lorraine—rarely, thankfully—at social events, I initially tried to avoid her, but eventually I treated her like the human she was, full of flaws and finding her way, but not Satan's mistress.

I got to the point where I smiled and hugged her hello. I would briefly endure the Lorraine Show until someone—please someone?—rescued me. It was common knowledge that Lorraine was like a radio on transmit 90 percent of the time, but she was tolerable, even entertaining, in small doses. Then, I would sincerely wish her well. Her life had not been easy, and I tried to exercise more empathy than distaste. If Eric wanted to communicate with her periodically, I would not object. He viewed it as a personal favor when I was cordial to her in person, and I liked to see him happy. It took only a small effort to swallow the snark and be pleasant for a few minutes.

That said, I would not have minded if I never saw her again for the rest of my life.

6.

Judgment-Free Zone

During the time Eric was dating Lorraine, I started therapy to manage stress and the temper that I had struggled with on and off for much of my adult life. My short fuse was a source of discord with Eric, whose anger was a slow burn coupled with an elephantine memory. I was in the passive-aggressive camp, sniping, "Am I the only one who sees the trash needs to be emptied?" Once my ire was out of my system, I was ready for makeup sex. Eric, on the other hand, needed at least two days to speak to me with anything other than disdain and distrust after my criticism had reared its head, believing my comments telegraphed intolerable contempt for him.

I hoped to find a calm, judgment-free environment for one hour a week to develop strategies to manage stress. Considering myself more practical than passionate, I consulted an expert in my personal life just as I hired experts to testify in court. I pictured my therapist as an infinitely patient, underweight, bearded guru sitting cross-legged in a cream-colored robe and hemp sandals. I would lay out my expectations and let the guru guide me.

The discouragingly short list of therapists who accepted my insurance and met on weekends to accommodate working moms led me to Ingrid. She was middle-aged, divorced, and working out of her home. As I sat silently in her living room on the claw-footed sofa of a forgettable color, staring at the lone picture of a bird on a branch, and waited my turn, I felt despair hang heavily in the air.

I did not relate well to Ingrid, although I was not sure how much I was supposed to. I viewed her as a technician for the limited purpose of helping me apply methodologies to make me calmer and more patient.

After a handful of sessions, I started to think I should tell her I was in an open marriage, even though it was not the reason for my sessions. Maybe she would find that information useful in helping me with my problem of catapulting from stoic to shrew in frustrated outbursts that had long predated my forays into non-monogamy and strained my relationship with Eric.

My feeling that I was being dishonest to my own detriment came to a head when I was dealing with some unpleasant Lorraine issue that left me teary-eyed right before driving to see Ingrid. I arrived feeling like there was an elephant in the room that only I could see. It was sitting on the claw-footed sofa staring at me via the cut-through window between Ingrid's office and waiting area, one eyebrow arched. (Do elephants have eyebrows?)

Really, Natalie? You don't think your therapist needs to know that your husband dates other women, that you are okay with the general principle, but that you cannot stand Lorraine, even though you are falling over yourself trying? Don't you think that just maybe that adds to your everyday stress level, and your therapist would benefit from a fuller picture of your home life? C'mon girl. Out with it. She's a professional. She can deal. Point taken, pachyderm.

"Ingrid," I began, "To get a more complete picture of my life, you should know that I am in an open marriage. My husband has a girlfriend. We have rules, and we communicate about their relationship almost daily. To be clear, I am not here to discuss that. I am here seeking therapy to handle my anger management issues. At times, Eric's relationship with Lorraine will impact my state of mind and mood, so I felt you should know about it." I patted myself on the back. Now we could move on in full honesty. The elephant would be proud.

Oh, my well-meaning, ivory-tusked friend, you could not have been more wrong. After a few more sessions, I learned that I was a topic of conversation outside the walls of Ingrid's office.

"Natalie, I was discussing you with my therapist," she said. "She thinks your relationship choices are unhealthy and, frankly, abusive. My obligation is to you and your emotional welfare, so I must tell you I am very concerned."

Add a frown, headshaking, and a bit of—I kid you not—handwringing.

I was surprised to be discussed at Ingrid's therapy session. I felt myself tense, but I refrained from saying, *Correct me if I am wrong, but I thought therapists were supposed to be nonjudgmental and accepting of alternative lifestyles. My husband didn't force me into this. I don't feel emotionally abused. In fact, opening up our marriage, as a whole, has been more positive than negative. Although, yes, it's a frakking roller coaster of emotions sometimes, we are working through it together, which strengthens our connection.*

I tried not to get angry and defensive. Maybe therapy was working.

I also did not say, *Ingrid, according to Dr. Geri Weitzman's 36-page pamphlet, "What Psychology Professionals Should Know About Polyamory," most poly people seek therapy for non-poly reasons. So, Inge—may I call you Inge?—you don't need to be a polyamory expert to be my therapist or to have an understanding that I am not an aberration worthy of a "Natalie" category in the DSM.*

What I did say, in my best therapist-speak, using the more moderate voice that was indicative of the improved impulse control she had helped me achieve, was a version of this. "Ingrid, I understand what you are feeling. I empathize that you may have no reference point to evaluate my lifestyle choice. I acknowledge that the dynamic I chose can be challenging, but it can also be rewarding."

I admitted that my open marriage added stress to my life, but, on balance, it added love and connection and moved me toward accepting Eric's whole self.

I considered what to do. I could find another counselor. Typically, those who identified as LGBTQIA+-friendly were also more poly-friendly, but I would have had to pay out of pocket since my insurance did not cover them.

I could stop counseling altogether, but I was reluctant to abandon what had been hard enough for me to start. I had benefited from the suggested breathing exercises and meditations to center myself each day.

I chose a third option. I decided to give her a chance to help me. When she broached my open relationship during a session, I answered briefly and redirected her to address my anger management.

However, the tenor of her disapproval became increasingly off-putting. It got to the point where I thought, *Look, lady, I am generally happy, healthy, successful, and sexually fulfilled. Can you say that? Is your monogamist outlook working for you and your cat?*

I also thought, *I can accept that different folks have different relationship preferences. Why can't you? I am struggling enough on my own to make sense of polyamory, and you are not helping my stress level. There are no roadmaps. There are no romance novels, Disney plots, or even Grimm fairy tales that tell how the princess grew up to have more than one loving and intimate relationship that fulfilled her and how she raised her children to appreciate that having more than one love did not make you less.*

After a period of weeks when one or both of us were unavailable, our sessions came to an end. I had probably gotten all I could from our relationship, and I figured she was relieved to be shed of me and my strange marital ways. Fortunately, I could talk to Eric about her and the counseling. After more than two decades, he knew me better than anyone.

I found it disheartening that not all therapists were educated or even well-read enough to help clients in open relationships. Such a deficiency in the counseling business was a disservice to non-monogamists. If I had been able to find a therapist who understood and accepted polyamory, I could have trusted them more, and ultimately, therapy for stress management, and how poly-management issues interacted and affected those, could have been more productive.

I am hopeful that as polyamorists come out of the closet and therapists encounter them more often, polyamory will become part of the counseling curriculum, just as counseling the LGBTQIA+ community on life issues has been. My sessions with Ingrid were more than ten years ago, and I understand from poly friends and acquaintances that the therapy profession has gotten better at addressing the needs of non-monogamists, especially as polyamorists become life coaches and counselors. Business is booming! One local therapist I knew had to limit her poly clients when she realized that more than one was in the same polycule.

Who knows? Maybe I have a potential second career as a poly-friendly therapist. The marketplace is calling.

PART TWO

7.
Starting with Friends

During the final year of Lorraine, I was faced with a health issue and doubts about my marriage. Maybe the Lorraine experience was the first step to separating or even divorce. I tried to read the polyamory instructional books, but some of them made me angry, and others bored me. I didn't feel like buying what they seemed to be selling. Was I supposed to rewrite my wedding vows, going from exclusive love and lifetime commitment to some flavor of 1960s free love? That did not sound like me, like us.

Some polyamory practices made sense to me. Coupled with Eric's explanation of how he viewed this relationship structure, the beginnings of my poly philosophy were forming. However, I did not consider myself polyamorous. I tolerated it, but I was not participating in it myself. I acknowledged and appreciated that Eric felt this relationship dynamic suited him, but I was still not so sure polyamory was right for me.

In addition to considering whether being in a polyamorous marriage was what I wanted physically and emotionally, we also faced the danger that public knowledge of a non-monogamous lifestyle could endanger our livelihoods. As a military officer, Eric was subject to the Uniform Code of Military Justice and could be prosecuted for adultery under Article 134, known as the General Article. The maximum punishment for adultery was a dishonorable discharge, forfeiture of all pay and allowances, and confinement for one year. We were aware of cases where penalties had been imposed, even though all parties were adults engaged in *consensual* non-monogamy. It required little foresight to predict a poly-unfriendly commander deciding that other service members knowing that their fellow soldier, aviator, marine, or sailor had a spouse *and* a lover—even if their spouse also had a lover—was, in the language of the General Article, a "discredit to the armed forces or had engaged in conduct prejudicial to good order and discipline." We can't have people enjoying sex with anyone but their spouses. That would be criminal.

Furthermore, I was employed in a public-facing legal job where I was bound by a broad ethics rule that made me subject to disciplinary action for engaging in what was vaguely described as conduct "prejudicial" to my employer. In a mandatory training session, when I asked our ethics officer what that meant, he was unsure.

Without outing myself to the roomful of colleagues, I pressed, "Would that cover adultery, for instance?"

"If it was illegal, then yes," he said. "Criminal acts would be grounds for discipline."

Since adultery was a misdemeanor where I lived, albeit rarely enforced, I kept silent. I knew from my research that consent was not an element of adultery in any of the dozen states that had not repealed it. It was still a felony in a few states, including Wisconsin, where Section 944.16 made adultery punishable by a minimum of a year in prison. Adultery was defined as "(1) A married person who has sexual intercourse with a person not the married person's spouse; or (2) A person who has sexual intercourse with a person who is married to another."

Violation of the law did not require a lack of consent by the allegedly aggrieved party. There was no requirement that the criminal offender have the mental state—the *mens rea*—to harm a non-consenting adult. The way adultery laws were written, it mattered not one iota whether the presumptively wronged spouse consented to the acts that constituted the crime. Thus, non-monogamists were considered adulterers—i.e., criminals—under the law.

Also at risk were poly parents who were employed at a conservative organization, a government agency, or a school, or a polyamorist with an estranged or former spouse prepared to use polyamory to allege parental unfitness in a custody battle. We had to be aware of the potential impact of our polyamory choices.

Eric deployed to Iraq a few months after the breakup with Lorraine. I had been accepted for a one-year position that did not require travel. A month before Eric left, I was diagnosed with breast cancer after a routine mammogram. A small piece of my breast was removed, and I had eight weeks of radiation. I took the train to the treatment center before work each day, and then the train to my office. I told three close friends, my sister, and my father. No one at work knew. Besides it being uncomfortable to wear a bra after a few weeks of radiation, there were no significant changes to my life. (I am fine now, thanks.)

I was essentially a single parent to a middle schooler while Eric was deployed. Will and I saw Eric on Skype once every week or two, depending on how our schedules aligned.

Even though as a headquarters officer, Eric's deployment was technically voluntary, it was, in all fairness, his turn. If he did not go, someone else would have had to. I understood that. I looked forward to the time apart to figure out some things, not the least of which was what was happening to my marriage.

Before Eric left, he said, "Just because I've decided to take this deployment does not mean you have to be alone. You can date. I want you to." He suggested friends and past swinger partners. He asked a mutual poly friend to come over and start his motorcycle periodically, as well as his wife.

"I am not you, Eric," I said. "I don't want that." I did not have the time, energy, or desire.

I kept myself busy with work, parenting, and radiation treatments. I had almost constant anxiety about whether Eric and I would be together when he came home. His emails too often felt rote or obligatory. I combed each line for signs of affection. I cried on my walks to and from the train, where Will could not witness it. The cancer was minor, but having been tagged with it made me feel like a weakling, a victim. I hated that feeling. I could not talk to Eric about any of it. He deployed before my first radiation treatment.

I imagined him thinking, *That's all I need, a sick wife.* Not that he ever said anything close to that, but our relationship was under strain. To be fair, he had been my rock during the surgery, steady and strong.

Then he was gone, oceans away amid life-threatening situations he did not share with me. I was alone.

After a few months on my own, I reached out to an old friend and one-time swinger partner whom Eric knew and respected. Vincent was my confidant in this poly transition. I had cried to him about Lorraine. He had reassured me I was not going insane, that my struggles with this new chapter of my life were normal, that yes, Eric loved me, and I was valuable and attractive and intelligent, and all the vain affirmations I desperately needed to hear. He and I had developed a close friendship, without the "benefits."

I had not had sex with anyone since Eric had been deployed, and I was starting to miss the intimacy. Vincent's current girlfriend lived on the West Coast, so they had agreed that Vincent could occasionally date separately.

On a bracing winter evening, I prepared to meet Vincent. As I showered, carefully shaved and perfumed myself, I felt like a temptress from a paperback romance novel. I rolled my eyes and took a breath. *Relax, Natalie. This is Vincent. You've had sex with him before.*

Standing naked in my bedroom, I felt liberated from my everyday beige bra and sensible cotton panties. From the back of my dresser drawer, I fished out a black push-up bra and a lacy scarlet and ebony thong. I held the skimpy lingerie to the light, checking for dust. None visible, I slid them on, hoping to also slide into a ready-for-action polyamorist persona.

Standing before the mirror as I pulled on a plunging V-neck sweater, the effect enhanced by the push-up bra, and zipped up a form-fitting skirt, I pictured Eric's grin and heard his decades-old compliment that I shrugged off as husbandly obligation: "Your ass is as perfect as the first time I saw it."

I could also imagine him saying to my reflective dismissal, "Natalie, if you don't believe me that you're hot, how about believing that fit and savvy tech guy, ten years your junior, waiting for you?"

I sucked in my gut and grabbed my keys. Driving across town, I buzzed with nervous excitement. I could feel my body becoming aroused as I imagined an evening alone with Vincent. I cracked the car window to tamp the flush that was rising.

For the first time, it would be just the two of us. No girlfriend, no husband. No worries about whether Eric was vibing with Vincent's partner or whether Vincent and I were gelling more or getting ahead of Eric along the road to fruition. I knew Vincent and I had sexual chemistry, but it had been a few years since we had been naked together as part of a swinger scenario with Eric and Vincent's prior local girlfriend.

At a stoplight, I reapplied lip gloss and messaged Vincent.

"ETA ten minutes."

"Be waiting in five" was his response.

I pulled into a parking spot and squirmed in the driver's seat to adjust the creeping thong. I saw Vincent grinning at me from outside the passenger side window. I startled.

"Hey, cutie," he said, smiling. "Didn't mean to scare you. I didn't want you out here in the dark alone."

In the hallway outside his apartment, I had a flashing fantasy of Vincent pushing me against the wall and ravishing me. Why was a bodice-ripping romance novel script playing in my brain? I hadn't read one since high school!

I declined his offer of alcohol. I was too heady already, high on this new experience of a one-on-one encounter. We sat on the sofa with our sodas, my boots shed and my bare feet tucked under me. I had trouble meeting Vincent's gaze. He seemed relaxed, while I was vibrating with the anticipation of skin-on-skin contact.

Without a word, Vincent took my hand and led me to the bedroom. He backed me to the bed, and I fell on it with a laugh. The laugh broke the spell and reminded me, *You've got this. Have fun.*

All pretense gone, he kissed me. I responded eagerly, hungrily. I had not held Eric in three months, and my body reacted to Vincent's touch like brittle paper to a match. We found our rhythm without much trouble, and after mutual satisfaction, there were mutual smiles.

Vincent's fingers trailed down the space between my breasts, and his lips brushed mine.

"You have no idea how amazing you are," he said.

I felt myself blush. "Right back at you."

The comfort of a friend—a sexy friend—had been the next step I needed in my open marriage journey. When I emailed Eric that I had been with Vincent, he was happy I was forging my own path. He wrote, "Do it because you like it, not to please me. As I have said many times, I like to hear about it. Even better, I would like to see it in naughty detail, but I know that you have always been uncomfortable talking about sex and are camera shy."

Vincent and I connected a few times over the next several weeks, but he had limited permission to date separately from his girlfriend. I understood this. They weren't polyamorous. They were swingers. She was granting us a dispensation because of the miles that separated her from Vincent and me from Eric.

Vincent and I remained friends, but we ended our sexual relationship after our window of permission closed. I continued to rely on his perspective, and I looked forward to sharing a meal and talking about our lives. Vincent was genuine about who he was, volunteering during his employer's security clearance process that he was a swinger even though no question asked, "Do you swing? If not, stop here. If yes, continue because we have a lot more questions for you, pervert."

The cost of Vincent's revelation to his employer that he was a swinger was submitting to a three-hour session with a psychologist. I think Vincent helped spread the non-monogamy gospel by telegraphing, *Hey, look at me, doc. I'm just a regular guy. I'm stable, educated, fully employed, with a girlfriend, a family I care about, and no criminal record. And, yes, I engage in a form of consensual non-monogamy called swinging.* I was in awe. I wished I dared to shout my relationship status from the rooftops, but I did not, at least not then.

I worried that I dumped too much of my relationship angst on Vincent, especially when Eric was seeing Lorraine, but he seemed to enjoy our discussions, active listener and problem-solver that he was. Because he knew me and my journey, his insights were valuable. Friends like Vincent were the icing on the poly cake. I could not imagine a world where we were not friends, even when we did not see each other for long periods. At that time, he was one of only a few poly friends I could talk to. Being polyamorous felt like a dirty secret.

During Eric's deployment, I moved along in my solo poly journey with one other friend. He and his wife were polyamorous. We four had been intimate together, and Eric had already suggested I connect with him. With each sexual experience independent of Eric, I moved closer toward polyamory, but I was not fully there yet. I existed in an in-between space, a limbo without a label. I didn't know if I was practicing situational polyamory because Eric was deployed, or if he and I would continue to date separately and form separate romantic relationships when he came home.

It was all too much to decide when I was unsure how Eric and I would sync as a couple when he returned after a year of separation. Although he had been in the military in some form since high school, the deployment was his first one. It was the first time we had been apart for more than a few weeks since our marriage.

I took more steps toward polyamory. My Canadian friend from the gym, Brooke, and I celebrated her birthday with lunch at a restaurant with a low decibel rating, curries popping with flavor, and seamless service. We chatted generally about workouts, our kids, and her new job.

When dessert arrived, she told me she was considering opening up her marriage. She asked me if I knew kink-friendly resources. I listened and tried not to appear as shocked as I felt. We had never discussed sex or open relationships.

I tried to act cool. *Well . . . I've heard of this site . . . I understand that this venue might be of interest, but I don't know myself.* I told her I had a friend she could contact who was more plugged into that scene. I made no personal admissions, and she sought none. I felt like a visitor to an alternate reality where neighborhood moms discussing sexual non-monogamy and bondage was typical lunch chat.

A week later I learned she had not only contacted my friend about her BDSM questions, but that they had hooked up. *That was fast work.* When we became closer as friends, as seemed inevitable, I asked her why in the world she had pegged me as someone receptive to her very personal questions, especially when I knew she was hyper-protective of her privacy.

"Some of your offhand comments made me suspect. You said you had a rule that Eric couldn't have sex with your housemate," Brooke said.

"That was a joke!" I said.

Maybe I was jonesing so much for a friend to talk to that I was hoping someone would figure it out. Later, I became less didactic about consciously separating friends who knew we were poly from those who did not.

Brooke and her husband had opened up their marriage based partially on their sexual incompatibility. He was submissive and a masochist in bed, meaning he liked a dominant to take control during sex and inflict pain for his pleasure.

"I can totally see you in a dominatrix outfit," Brooke said with a grin. "I think you would be a great sexual match for my husband. I've told him about you." Because of my goth wardrobe, I had the clothes for the role. Curious about whether I could pull off being a Domme, I accepted her invitation to try it with her husband.

Not until after donning form-fitting leather from boots to bodice did I discover how I felt dominating him physically. I had no experience with a Dominant/submissive or D/s dynamic other than light play I saw at dance clubs where someone, usually a woman, might be spanked or lightly flogged in a dark corner as part of the taboo aesthetic. I paid little attention to it.

With Brooke's husband, I learned that I abhorred inflicting pain, even though he wanted me to. I naively had imagined that wielding a riding crop would be exciting role-play, like a saucy wench who turned the tables on a rakish stranger. Instead, I winced, desperately wanting to turn my face from him each time I heard the thwacking sound of my leather staff as it landed on his flesh and saw the pink trails on his pale skin.

Before each stroke I asked in a fearful whisper, "Is that okay?" and he responded, "Yes, but you can go harder," when I wanted him to say he had had enough, so we could enjoy each other's bodies without props. I might have been a no-nonsense, analytic attorney during the day, but I didn't want to walk over anyone, in spiked heels or otherwise, at night.

Also at Brooke's invitation, I had sex with her new boyfriend, who was a stranger to me and remained so. As part of their dominant (him) and submissive (her) power dynamic, her boyfriend instructed her to find a woman for him to satisfy while Brooke waited in the next room, listening to the sounds of pleasure or pain, to demonstrate his dominance and her submission to his will.

I agreed to spare my friend from trolling for a woman on Craigslist to complete her assignment. I also was curious about this man she described as a fantastic lover. However, I knew from photos she had shown me that I did not find him physically attractive. I insisted on being blindfolded during the entire encounter, in part to keep distance between us, in part to add danger and fun, and frankly, so I could fantasize about what I wished he looked like.

He was a good lover, but I later found out that he had instructed Brooke to watch us in bed, and she had silently crept to the doorway despite my insistence that I was not game for that kind of voyeurism. She apologized, but that was the last time I helped her with any submissive task.

I had explored sex with friends. I had explored sex with my friend's husband and with her lover. I had not ventured out completely on my own to meet someone new by myself. The prospect terrified me. It also thrilled me.

8.
Polyfuckery?

There were two dance clubs where I felt comfortable going without Eric. I knew some of the regular crowd, and I felt safe enough to dance, have a drink, and talk to friends. On the few occasions I went out while Eric was in Iraq, it took an abundance of self-talk to push myself out the door. I was able to have a night out because we had taken on a boarder, who helped out in the same manner as Helen had. Since he was home most nights studying for his graduate program, he could monitor Will, granting me relief from middle school homework marathons and solo parenting.

I knew Will would be safe. He played video games and read Harry Potter, his beloved dog curled up at his side. Before leaving, I always reminded Will that I had my cell phone if he needed me. He would smile and say, "You look pretty, Mom."

On a Saturday six months into Eric's deployment, a small dance club we had been to many times hosted a pirate-themed night. I coveted an opportunity to dress (hide behind?) the theme. I printed two Jolly Roger line drawings I found online and carefully sewed the paper images onto the triangles of a black bikini top. I draped a black scarf around my hips and secured it with a chunky black belt from Eric's closet that had metal links in the shape of skulls crossed with swords. I pulled on black fishnets and tall black boots.

Not bad, I thought as I looked in the mirror. *Try to suck in your stomach.* I belted a trench coat before saying good night to Will and drove to the familiar venue, mentally reminding myself to only have one drink.

At the club, I willed myself to walk across the parking lot.

C'mon, Natalie, you can do this. You've been to this club a dozen times. You can leave any time.

I walked through the alley and up the stairs, wiping my palms on my coat. I flashed my driver's license, paid the cover charge, and surrendered the inside of my wrist for a bat-shaped ink stamp.

The brick three-story structure was an artist workspace during the day. The familiar smell of aerosol finishing spray hung on the air in the stairwell. When I walked inside the club, I was relieved to see friends and hear familiar music. I felt the deejay's set cleanse me of the work week as I danced, my eyes closed, my head swaying. After a few songs, with a light sweat starting, I sipped a drink from the bar while watching others dance. I breathed deeply, trying to surrender to the night.

In line for the restrooms, I heard, "I like what you're wearing. Very thematic." A dark-haired guy with biceps straining under his short-sleeved shirt was grinning at me and my bikini top.

"Thanks," I said. "The wonders of the internet and a printer." The restroom door opened, and I went in.

Later, as I was resting on a bench and drinking water, the same guy asked to sit next to me. He told me it was his first time at the club, but he knew a few of the same people I did and liked the music. I went back to the dance floor. Wasn't that why I was there? Yes, but also. . . .

He was attractive and perhaps interested in me. I realized that not only was I lonely for male company, but that I was allowed to act on my feelings, even with someone Eric didn't know.

Sometime later, the guy caught my attention again. "Hey, I just wanted to say good night. It was really nice talking with you. My friends are leaving, so I have to go with them since they're my ride."

I asked where he lived. It wasn't on my way home, but it wasn't that far out of the way. His politeness and clean-cut vibe made him seem non-threatening. I would be the one driving, not him. My heart rate spiked at the possibility of what the night could bring.

I decided to take a chance. "I drove, so if you want to stay longer, I could take you home."

"Are you sure?"

"It's no problem."

In the car, I noticed a tribal pattern tattoo on his left shoulder. "Any other tattoos?" I asked.

"No, but I have a piercing that you can't see when I have my pants on."

"Oh?" I had heard of such piercings but had never seen one, let alone felt one.

"Yeah, it's a rod, like a barbell. I thought it would intensify sex." He shrugged. "I don't know if it does though."

I wouldn't mind collecting data and making my own conclusion, I thought, gripping the steering wheel. *This ride just became more interesting.*

When we reached his apartment, I parked with the building entrance on the driver's side. He said, "Thanks for the ride. That was really sweet of you." He started walking toward the building.

I had never given a man I had just met a ride home from a club. In the movies, the guy always asked the girl up. Was he being polite? Waiting for my move? Not that interested? Tired?

I didn't know the protocol in real life, but I was not about to let him slip through my fingers, after I had worked up the nerve to get as far as I had, without making some kind of move.

I lowered the driver's side window. "I could come up if you want."

"Yeah? You sure it's not too late?"

"It's not too late for me."

His apartment was sparsely furnished. It had no couch, and the only decor was a wall map with push pins of places he had been. Had he just moved in? He offered me a drink, and we talked about travel.

He apologized for the state of the apartment. "I work a lot."

After what seemed like forever, but was probably thirty minutes, of no physical contact but plenty of electricity in the space between us, I wondered if he was ever going to kiss me. He had not asked me to leave. He had not said he needed to be up early. What was I missing?

I closed the distance between us and stood on my tiptoes, my face even with his. I placed my hands lightly on his muscular shoulders, slowly took his lips in mine, and closed my eyes. He kissed me back, holding me close enough that I could feel that he was interested.

"Do you want to show me your bedroom?" I asked.

He smiled. "Yes."

We undressed each other, and I admired his taut chest and round biceps. I traced my finger along his arm tattoo. When I lowered his boxer briefs, I tried not to stare at the piercing.

When he untied my bikini top, and I let it drop to the floor, he breathed, "You're gorgeous."

On the bed, he shimmied down until he was looking up from my knees.

"Is this okay?" he asked.

"Yes," I smiled and thought, *Thanks for asking.*

I asked if he had a condom, and he fished one from a drawer.

Despite vigorous and repeated engagement, I did not feel his piercing. Perhaps more data was necessary.

After I was dressed and ready to leave, he said apologetically, "I had a lot to drink tonight. Maybe we can try this again soon? I'd like to bring my A game."

I felt obtuse. I had chalked up his failure to climax to first-time nerves. I then realized that maybe that was why he had not pounced on what I thought was my obvious flirting. I wasn't tracking how much he drank at the club. He was not unsteady or slurring.

Eric didn't drink much. I could not recall a time when his arousal or performance had been affected by alcohol. It had not occurred to me that my much younger, pierced lover might have labored under suboptimal conditions.

"That would be great," I said. "I had a nice time." We exchanged cell numbers and a deep goodbye kiss that left me flushed.

The highway was mostly deserted. For at least half of the ten miles home, I nearly bounced in my seat, full of euphoric energy, as I said aloud over and over, like a mantra I could not stop, "I cannot fucking believe I just did that. I cannot fucking believe it."

I wanted to scream out the window, *I took a hot guy home, and we had sex!*

I wanted to tell Eric, several time zones to the east, *You will never guess what I just did! What a thrill!*

As I neared my house, where my son and housemate would be asleep, I told myself to calm down.

Breathe, girl.

Yes, for the first time in your life, you took a guy back to his place, had sex with him, and lived to tell the tale. Maybe not the safest course of action, but I understand the excitement. The rawness of it. You never did that in your twenties or thirties. Now you know what it's like. Welcome to the Slut of the Month Club.

Now, chill.

Proud of my restraint, I waited a whole three days to text him.

"Friday night was fun. I will take you up on your offer of a repeat. When works for you?"

I didn't hear from him that day, or for a few days after. He said he worked a lot, so maybe he was busy. I waited another couple of days and texted again.

"Hey, there. I hope you're having a good week. I could come over this Friday or Saturday. Let me know if that works or if another day is better."

The next day came his reply. "Hey. Sorry, this weekend I am out of town. I don't know when my schedule will open up. I'll try to find a time."

For another week, I held out hope, but all I got was silence. Then I got irritated. Then I was deflated, realizing that I was not going to hear from him again. That was another first for me—a one-night stand.

Was that how it went?

I didn't know how hookups and dating worked. I had little experience with dating, since Eric and I became exclusive when I was nineteen. I tried to put a bright face on the experience despite my disappointment. I took a chance, had some fun, and that was that. What would be the next step in my dating and sexual evolution sans Eric?

Little by little I was branching out on my own. It was mainly sex; not really what I considered dating. I was not having the kind of fuller relationship Eric had with Lorraine, but I was getting out there. I was experiencing some of the validation and thrill that I supposed was what attracted Eric to polyamory. I was moving outside the swinging format, but I didn't know if it was polyamory. Some might have called it polyfuckery.

Polyfuckery was explained to me as having sex with multiple partners without much if any emotional attachment or relationship component. The term may have been intended to have a negative connotation by polyamorists who prioritized love and commitment over sexual connection and who could be quick to remind the great unwashed that poly*amory* refers to love, so if you were not in love, you were doing polyamory wrong.

While my snarky instinct might have been to roll my eyes and shout *Embrace your inner slut!*, I recognized that different interactions had varying levels of connection. My experience with swinging, for example, entailed a low level of attachment. However, I knew swingers who had sex with other couples as well as caught baseball games together and had cookouts with their kids.

I saw the emotional value of multidimensional relationships that contained more tender feelings. Eric and Lorraine had those feelings for each other.

It came down to the soup question. If you were sick in bed, would your partner schlep to your place and deliver soup and sympathy? That demonstrated a level of commitment and caring potentially absent in polyfuckery.

Eric was my soup person. He was my love and support. I wondered if I needed or wanted that level of emotional involvement with someone else, or even multiple someones. Maybe polyamory was a relationship structure that embodied a sliding scale of commitment and attachment.

I was not sure if polyamory was what I wanted for myself long-term, or if it was more of a placeholder while Eric was away. He was jubilant that I was taking these steps, but I downplayed them in my emails to him. I thought of my actions more as occupying myself while I was alone. I didn't have a boyfriend, and I was not looking for one. I was having some fun experiences, but was that polyamory? From what I had read, what I was doing was more like hooking up with my husband's permission.

I didn't know then that on a steamy July evening, six weeks before Eric was to fly home, I would discover that polyamory for me was not just sex. It was connection, it was addictive, and as Janet sang to Rocky, I wanted more, more, more.

9.

A New Start

Eric had not taken any leave in the nine months he had been deployed, and he was entitled to some R&R. Through email, our primary mode of communication, he sent me a proposal for using his two weeks of vacation in June. For the first week, he would join Lorraine at a festival of the dark music they both liked. For the second week, he would meet me on the Spanish island of Ibiza, since he knew how much I loved the beach.

My relationship with Eric had been so strained while he was away that I was pleasantly surprised to be included in his plans at all. I accepted the Lorraine part of the vacation equation. During Eric's deployment, Lorraine sent him novels and helped keep his spirits up, and I did not begrudge him that comfort.

To meet him in June, I placed Will with two different households. I hated to impose on the parents of Will's friends, but I assuaged my guilt by knowing that Will was a well-behaved kid and that the parents seemed genuine in their offers to help me facilitate a reunion with Eric.

My mom friends were generous in their support of my vacationing with my absent husband. They didn't know Eric was seeing his lover the week before meeting me. They didn't know about our lifestyle, as far as I knew anyway. I was not overly concerned that my neighborhood friends would shun me, but I could not control their dissemination of information and ensure it would not end up embarrassing my son, who didn't know yet, and causing him pain, or compromising Eric's or my job security.

***

I landed in Ibiza an hour before Eric was due to arrive. In the baggage claim area where we had agreed to meet, I sat in a plastic airport chair that was attached to another plastic airport chair and waited.

My throat was dry. My palms were damp. My heart was thumping in stereo. I had to pee, but I didn't want to risk missing him. Having to use the bathroom when I was nervous was routine for me, but I wasn't nervous. I was terrified.

I was terrified that Eric would greet me with the flat tone he used when he was angry with me and trying to get through an encounter. I was terrified that he had realized, after being apart from me and coming from a week of fun with Lorraine, that he did not love me and wanted a divorce. I was terrified that he would look at me with disdain, or even loathing, and wonder why he had stayed with an uptight, impatient, killjoy wife.

I remembered sitting across from him at the fancy restaurant I had booked for our twentieth wedding anniversary four months before his deployment.

"Maybe twenty years is long enough," he had said. I had willed my brimming eyes to focus on my appetizer and tried to unhear his words.

A year later, in the Ibiza airport, my right leg bounced incessantly. I tried self-talk.

Relax. If he didn't want to spend time with you, he wouldn't have invited you. Run away with Lorraine? Please. She may be fun, but she is not run-away-and-live-together fun. You'll be okay no matter what happens. You will figure it out and survive. He proposed a vacation he knew you would enjoy. Sun, sand, nightclubs. That says something.

Thankfully, his plane was a little early or I might have Rumpelstiltskin'd my leg through the linoleum floor. I heard his flight announced and kept my eye on the Arrivals door. I made myself take deep, slow breaths as I stared straight ahead.

The man I had loved for more than half my life, tall and lean, his sand-colored, Army-issue backpack slung over one shoulder, his face serious, his eyes scanning for me, had arrived. I squinted at his short hair. Had he gone completely gray in the past year?

I dared a tight smile and stood. I waited for him to see me, preparing myself for whatever reaction might come.

He saw me and grinned. I walked to him.

He wrapped me in his arms, and we kissed. The tender warmth of his lips against mine filled me with emotion. I felt my chest heaving. I fought back tears, but a few leaked out. I withdrew from the kiss and brushed at my wet cheeks.

"You look good," he said.

"So do you," I said carefully. "Your hair seems lighter."

"Do you like it? It's my Billy Idol look," he said. "I had a layover in Kuwait and had it dyed. They didn't do the best job." He shrugged. "You always said I should try blond. I did it for you."

I was touched. "I love it."

Although Eric's hair was naturally dark brown like mine, I had seen photos of him as a tallow-haired toddler. With his skin tone, I always thought he would look good as a blond. I was right, and so was he. He reminded me of my favorite sexy '80s icon.

The music and movies of our college days were tightly woven into the tapestry of our relationship. We danced to Scandal, Joan Jett, and Madonna at nightclubs and drove to Austin for an outdoor Cars concert. That one of us could recite a movie line or sing a lyric and the other would grin and finish the quote or verse was just one of the threads that bound us in a way that he could not share with someone younger.

The stories Eric told at dinner parties were not just ones I had heard a dozen times, but ones I had lived. Like the time in college when he told me he was "fixin' to go to class."

I, his Yankee girlfriend, repeated, "You're *fixin'*?"

Eric would flash me a smile across the table and say, "I never said fixin' again."

"That's true." I would smile back. "He never did." We would both laugh.

We had lived a life together. We knew that the few weeks of summer stickiness the Washingtonians groused about were nothing compared to the routine 90-percent humidity of the Lone Star State. We were unshaken in our conviction that vinegary Carolina barbeque had nothing on the rich, smoky flavor of tender Texas brisket. We agreed that pints of Ben and Jerry's were poor substitutes for tubs of creamy Brenham-made Blue Bell ice cream, the frozen confection of our youth. When Eric worked at a convenience store in college, we passed a flat wooden spoon between us to finish off two-dollar pints of Homemade Vanilla.

Was our shared history all we had, and was twenty years "enough"? Our airport reunion gave me hope.

Most of our room in the beachfront Ibiza hotel was filled by the double bed, and it had a sliver-sized view of the azure Mediterranean. Eric loved rooms with a view; he had chosen a rooftop restaurant with a view of the US Capitol for our wedding rehearsal dinner. By the time we had stowed our luggage and hung up a few items to stave off further wrinkling, it was eight o'clock in the evening.

"Spaniards eat dinner late, so there's no rush," Eric said.

I looked into his eyes. I found no hint of animosity, but I was still afraid to assume anything. Our last intimate encounters before his deployment had at times been tense or fraught with unspoken hurts and expectations. How would sex be after so many months apart that had been filled with my trepidation about our future?

Eric cupped my face tenderly in his hands. His touch warmed me, as it always had. He kissed me gently and deeply. I slowly savored him. He tasted like home and history, like love and lust. My body temperature rose, responding with muscle memory. Our bodies moved together effortlessly, and we slid against and within each other. Eric beamed at me, his face full of affection and joy. I began to wonder if I had imagined an awkward estrangement before and during his deployment that had made me question if we would be together when he came home.

My release was physical and emotional. I nuzzled my head into Eric's chest and silently sobbed with relief. Yet, I was not confident enough to fully let go of my anxiety. I would see where the week took us. I committed to listening, being open, and enjoying each other and the days ahead on the island.

We had four days together in the Fort Lauderdale of Europe. We spent our days sunning on the sand. We ate lunch in the late afternoon at cafes on the beach, disco-napped, and made love before dinner. We savored Spanish dinners at ten o'clock and were dancing at the clubs by midnight, which was early for Spaniards. We tried to stay out late enough to see the tiered dance floor of one club fill with water like a swimming pool, but we called it quits at 3:00 a.m. We were at the club long enough to see aerialists swing over our heads and acrobats contort to the electronic music and gleeful shouts of club patrons. I was delighted that Eric had researched to find this indoor amusement park for adults.

Eric admired the magenta bikini I had bought for the trip. "You're so sexy," he said, beaming. "I've missed you, Natalie."

I blushed. "That's nice to hear."

I thought but did not say, *I was so afraid that you wouldn't feel that way, that you didn't love me anymore. I've lived in fear for months. I used to tell you my every emotion and want to know yours, but these past two years, a wall has seemed to grow, brick by brick. What are you feeling now? What do you see for us?*

It seemed dangerous to light that fuse, to potentially ruin our vacation with reality. We had only a few days together. When our island getaway was over, he was headed back to Iraq to complete the last weeks of his assignment. I flew back home, our home.

I wrote to Eric:

> Thanks so much for an unparalleled vacation of pure sloth: sex, sun, sand, sangria, suds, sushi, steak, sex [oh, did I already mention that?]. It was so great to see you, and I enjoyed our time together. A lot. And often.
>
> And . . . [is it hot in here?] I am an Ibiza fan and will be recommending it to everyone. :)

He responded with gratitude, his top love languages being words of affirmation and physical touch:

> I'm really glad to hear that you had a good time in Spain. You seemed to, but it's nice and helpful to hear it from you explicitly. "Unparalleled"!
>
> Sounds like a ringing performance evaluation. I will take that. I thought it was fabulous as well. When things suck here I am going to visualize being on the beach in Ibiza.

After Ibiza, I was cautiously optimistic about my marriage and my connection to Eric. I felt that the twenty-pound weight that had been lying on my chest had been reduced to five. Eric had missed me. Perhaps not pined for me, but clearly we still loved each other, and I was encouraged we could find our way forward together.

10.

Failure to Appear

While Eric was deployed, my friend Brooke, who had recently opened her marriage, asked for my opinion on a dating profile she had created for a kink site called CollarMe.

Both she and her husband were more submissive than dominant on the BDSM spectrum, making their bedroom activities a constant challenge, each having to be the switch for the other because two bottoms (submissives) and two tops (dominants) did not make for a compatible kinky sexual dynamic. On the site, Brooke could find a master to leave her with the colorful bruises she wore with honor. Outside the bedroom, no one dominated Brooke, an accomplished professional, but behind closed doors was another matter.

Brooke asked me to take a look at her profile, but when I pulled up the URL, her profile did not appear. I surmised that I had to be a member to access the content, so I created a skeletal profile with a screen name and basic information like gender, age, and location. A photo was required, so I added one from my phone. It was a provocative even if G-rated photo of my torso, bare navel exposed, in the pink bikini I bought on a shopping trip with Brooke for my Ibiza vacation. On a lark, I had snapped the photo in the mall dressing room.

After I uploaded my profile, I was able to see Brooke's profile, and I considered my mission accomplished. However, I immediately received an alert that I had several messages from the site. Intrigued and surprised, I opened them. I read comments that made me blush, like "Nice abs" and "Hot!" The gist of the messages was, "So, what are you into?" and "What are you looking for?"

Those were good questions. I had never engaged in much self-examination in a kink context. I had worn latex dresses, fishnets, and a studded leather collar at a goth club for edgy effect, and I had danced at a club that had a spanking bench and a six-foot X-shaped wooden cross fitted with rings to attach wrist cuffs, known as a St. Andrews cross, but I did not participate. I went to the club to dance. I did not consider myself kinky.

After reading the list of kink classifications and activities a user could add to their profile, including many I had to look up and more than a few that made me grimace, I didn't know how to categorize myself. When I thought about what I wanted from a poly dating relationship, I wondered if CollarMe was a site worth exploring. I was not going to pick up guys at bars anymore, and I was not interested in dating my friends. Easing into polyamory with an old friend like Vincent had been like skiing the bunny slope. While I might not have been ready for black diamond runs, I was eager to explore something new.

I had little more than time to lose and potentially something not yet knowable to gain, so I filled in my profile. I checked a dozen boxes that asked what I liked kink-wise—rope, bondage, blindfolds, threesomes. I was largely winging it, having limited knowledge and even less experience. Considering the time that I spent looking up terminology, generating the profile took a while. I didn't know if I was dominant, submissive, or a switch. I knew from Brooke that a *switch* was someone who could be dominant or submissive, depending on the circumstances. But what were watersports? Hard limits? Cream pies? I was lost.

I gave my basic statistics: five foot six, 120 pounds, dark hair, hazel eyes, heterosexual, and female. The photo I uploaded provided a general idea of my physique without showing my face. I wrote, "I am in an open marriage and exploring this site. I don't know that I fall squarely into any kink category. I am not into intense pain."

After my Ibiza trip and less than two months before Eric was due home, I received an email notifying me that I had a message on the site.

I will never forget the effect the message had on me—the tone, the directness, the easy confidence without arrogance. The sender had posted a playful photo of himself goofing in a straw fedora. From the sliding glass refrigerator door in the photo's background, it looked like he had picked the hat off a rack at a gas station convenience store. He tipped the brim toward the camera and looked up from under it. He had intensely dark hair and eyes.

In a second photo, he was smolderingly sexy in a white bath towel wrapped provocatively around his waist. My eyes followed the hair on his toned chest down to the towel's edge. But really, it was what he said more than how he looked that did me in.

"It takes a lot to rise above the din on this site, and you do," messaged Felix. "I am looking for a visceral connection. You are stunning."

I agreed with him about the noise on the site. The messages I had received before his were either X-rated and gross or the generic "hey how ya doing," with little thought to their verbiage or response to the content of my profile, besides the photo of me in a bikini. As for "visceral," I found that word carnal and powerful. Words, they got me every time, and his were thoughtful, seemingly genuine, and flattering. They wooed me.

We talked late at night on the small chat box that popped up on my laptop. Flirting online was new to me. I found our exchanges easy, sexy, and fun. We traded movie links and dating experiences. I thought he had good taste in movies—because we had the same taste in movies. He was in the film and commercial production and postproduction business. He grasped editing and lighting nuances and geeked on backstories of films. I loved talking with him. He would ask what I liked about a film, and I would tell him without hesitation. We traded YouTube links to our favorite movie scenes. I felt heard.

After a week of chatting, our schedules meshed enough to meet at a bistro in my neighborhood on a steamy July evening. My local restaurant choice was potentially risky because a neighbor or a soccer mom who didn't know I was in an open marriage might see me with a man not my husband. These were women whose homes I walked to for holiday parties and with whom I chaperoned fourth-grade field trips to the Smithsonian. I had confided in them about illness and parenting and talked about sex and drugs and rock 'n' roll, shared recipes and gardening tips, and sipped red wine while our kids sorted Halloween candy after trick-or-treating. I wish I could have been an open book and shared my date excitement with my mom friends, especially while Eric was away, but, like many non-monogamous parents, I could not ignore the possibility that a neighbor or teacher would call child protective services.

That night, however, as I walked the half mile to meet Felix, I felt daring and flush with anticipation in my short cotton dress with thin shoulder straps, which zipped up the front. Felix wore a dark, form-fitting T-shirt, dark indigo jeans, and an engaging grin. We sat inches apart on the patio and drank red wine, our elbows on the table, leaning close to be sure to catch every word, every expression, every breath. We talked for hours about his history and mine, films, books, and music. We meshed on so much.

He leaned in close and said, "I want to kiss you now. I don't care who sees. Do you?"

My hands suddenly felt damp in my lap.

I shook my head and turned my chin to him.

When he kissed me, I felt heat shoot from my core to my red painted toes. I was sure I blushed, but thankfully it was too dark to see it, or at least I hoped. As we each drank our second glass of wine, I could feel it getting hotter outside, or maybe inside, under my dress, between my legs. The patio was full of patrons, but they were a blur of shadows in my periphery, outside our two-person bubble. We sat close as we talked, lowering our voices when we spoke of more intimate topics such as his past relationships with two women. Under the wrought iron table, my thigh brushed his, or maybe his brushed mine. Neither one of us moved away. When I inhaled, his scent filled my head. It wasn't cologne so much as an earthiness, a maleness.

He kissed me again, slowly, and said, "I already closed out the tab, so we can leave any time."

I nodded and said softly, "I'm ready to go."

"What do you want to do now?" he asked.

I blushed again and thought quickly. I was uncomfortable bringing him to my home after only one date, but I felt a powerful need for his skin against mine. The closest motel was within walking distance. I had driven by dozens of times but had never been inside. The Scotsman was a two-story affair with exterior walkways and doors I could see from the road. It looked like a place that rented rooms by the week.

"I know somewhere close," I said.

He drove to the motel and went inside to pay. I stayed in the car. I had no idea if that was what I was supposed to do. It was how I had seen women in the movies behave, the ones having affairs. I wasn't having an affair, but that was my single reference point. The only man I had ever checked into a hotel with was Eric. I barely recognized the woman lightly perspiring into my summer dress. Anticipation of his touch was heightened. Our online chatting had been candid, and the electricity I felt in person was so volatile I thought I might ignite like dry leaves in the path of a forest fire.

We were half a step inside the room when he slowly began to unzip my dress. I feared I would melt into a puddle, and the only evidence of me would be a wet spot on a threadbare carpet. I remained standing as he sat on a chair and tugged the metal toggle down between my breasts, past my waist to my hips.

As he pulled, he said, "I have been eyeing that zipper all night." The dress fell away, and I stepped out of it and my sandals. Besides my earrings, that's all I had on.

His mouth and hands were on me. I had read about people going at each other hungrily. I wouldn't have been surprised to find burns in the shape of his fingers and palms from where he touched me. We never turned on a lamp. We had knocked over the only one in the room, and it stayed that way. A streetlight cast shadows across the room.

After sex that left me breathless, Felix drove me the mile to an address I gave him, a block from my house. I waited until he pulled away and crossed two streets to walk home.

Felix had described himself as "always dominant" in his profile, and he delivered. He handled me with assurance but tenderness, discernibly skilled at eliciting pleasure from a partner. He was attuned to my every breath, body shift, and whimper. I gave myself to him without question. In retrospect, I realized my recklessness. When I told Eric about it later, he was shocked that I had unknowingly engaged in *breath play*, where air supply is briefly blocked, and the bottom may lose consciousness momentarily to enhance arousal. The hint of danger with Felix had been intoxicating, but after Eric's warning, I was ashamed of my carelessness and told Felix I had not consented and could not do that again.

"Natalie, you know I would never hurt you or put you at risk. I knew what I was doing. You were out for a second at most," he said. "But I understand."

I felt him seared into my flesh and psyche like a brand. I was surprised that it didn't bother me when I noticed minor bruising on my inner thighs and felt soreness the next day. No one had ever left deliberate marks on me.

I stood before my bathroom mirror examining the yellow, then greenish fingerprints on my skin. "To remind you of me," he responded when I lightly groused in a text about him marring my flesh. As if I needed a tangible souvenir to remember him, but hell if I was going to tell him that.

While Eric was deployed, I found it hard to fall asleep in an empty bed. I began staying up way too late and chatting online with Felix, who was a night owl. I was attracted to how he intuited my desires and flattered by how he seemed to crave me as much as I did him. He didn't overdo the compliments. A single word was enough. He had an urbane but not stuffy way about him. Although he was in his thirties to my forties, I felt that he could show me things, open my eyes as easily as he had opened my body.

He told me about a high-end lingerie shop in Manhattan where he had slipped the clerk cash for privacy with his girlfriend in the changing room. As a mental image of them formed, it changed, substituting me for her. The thought of Felix taking me in close quarters in a semi-public place excited me. I imagined him guiding me, patiently telling me in his deep, quiet voice exactly what to do in the small space, maneuvering my body under his hand to avoid me hitting my head or banging my elbow, his strong arms there to catch me or to pull me onto his lap as I tried to keep moans from escaping my mouth.

We saw each other a few more times in the next weeks. They were raw and intense encounters. Once, I offered up my wrists to be bound with the decorative hotel fabric strip that I found across the foot of the bed, and he obliged. Afterwards, as we dressed, he quietly stared at me.

"What?" I asked.

"I could really like you."

"Don't worry," I said, "you'll come to your senses soon enough." I smirked, as if my nonchalance could hide my intense feelings of *new relationship energy* or *NRE* that nearly buckled my knees. Eric had told me about the term used to describe that giddy, all-consuming feeling experienced in the initial stage of a romance.

Felix could make my face redden in public merely by raising an eyebrow or briefly touching the small of my back, as we followed a hostess to our table.

I was falling into a whirlwind of feelings at what we had and the possibilities of what that might become. Eric would be back in a matter of weeks. What would happen then? If we continued with our open marriage and Eric dated separately, then I too could date. I could date Felix and find out if the NRE was a spark that went out, or if he was a gateway to a wider world of visceral, multidimensional connection that reached my head and heart, as well as below my belt. Full-on polyamory.

Felix's job made planning dates almost impossible. He would tell me he wanted to see me, but he had a shoot, a West Coast phone call, or some work to finish, and he hoped to see me after, but was not sure what time. I interpreted that to mean we had a date, barring a work crisis. I kept the evening open and waited. And waited. Nine times out of ten, the shoot went long or there was a complication with a client, and we did not meet.

From his perspective, he never actually canceled on me. From my perspective, he kept me hanging all evening, like a fish on a line. I winced at not having my customary control. Felix taking control inside the bedroom was one thing—a delicious, desirable, and intense thing—but inside my head, while I was fully clothed and we were miles apart, was a horse of a different color. I saw red.

Our relationship, such that it was, began when I was rarely occupied by men other than Eric, so I rationalized that I was not giving up time with anyone else to wait for his call. However, the psychological toll was soul-crushing. I felt disregarded by a man I wanted to see so badly I ached. Later, when Eric returned home and was also dating, I often felt abandoned by what I viewed as Felix's broken dates or promises of dates when I could have made other plans while Eric was on his own date.

I vacillated between thinking Felix was playing me as part of a twisted dominant/submissive head game where he kept me emotionally naked on a leash of need and want, and that he was just as frustrated as I was at his inability to connect in person. The truth was probably somewhere closer to the latter. He was well aware that I did not like that treatment because I told him, repeatedly, with exasperation.

Years before we met, Felix had been in a *throuple* or *triad*, a relationship structure where each of the three members of the relationship has a romantic relationship with each other. In his case, he was in an intimate relationship with two bisexual women, and the women were in a sexual relationship with each other. If members of a triad do not have relationships outside of the triad, they are in a *closed* triad. Picture a triangle where each point is a relationship between the connecting lines.

A triad differs from a polyamorous *V* or *hinge* structure. Polyamory can be series of V formations with the hinge partner connecting each new V. In the Lorraine scenario, where Eric is the hinge of the V and I am one arm, if I date Felix, then I am the hinge in a new V with Eric as one arm and Felix as another. If Felix had more partners, he would be the hinge between me and someone else, and so on. The members of each V connected by a shared common hinge partner are members of a *polycule*, a term derived from molecule, where partners and metamours are the component atoms. In the above configuration, Lorraine, Eric, Felix, and I would be members of a polycule.

In some polycules, members have intimate relationships with partners of their partners' partners—whew—such as if Felix (my partner) had dated Lorraine (my partner Eric's partner). Welcome to the salacious polyamory that the mainstream media drools to write about and tag with a cover story photo of limbs intertwined in an orgiastic tangle under the covers of a king-sized bed. Usually, the duvet cover is a crisp white, and the toenails of at least one woman are scarlet.

I figured Felix would be better equipped to handle jealousy because he had been in a long-term polyamorous relationship, but he struggled from the outset. He later told me that he believed he could never have as much of me as he wanted. What he didn't seem to grasp, despite my telling him, was that he had me. When I was with him, I was his. Felix asked me if Eric's return meant that we would have to stop dating. It didn't, and I told him that.

Once home, Eric quickly became serious with a new girlfriend, Marianne, seeing her every week and talking with her every day. While Eric and I enjoyed a renewal of our emotional and physical relationship, we both pursued dating others. After my experiences with Vincent, Felix, and a few others, I was eager to find a steady partner like Eric had with Marianne. Eric encouraged my pursuits. I had anticipated that those pursuits would include Felix. I fantasized about all the fun we would have together, including overnights and weekend getaways. I thought he imagined the same. I couldn't have misread this, could I?

Instead of telling me what was going on with him, with us, Felix withdrew. At times, I thought I was being gaslit. A well-meaning friend, who had been burned by a cheater who had lied to her about being single, tried to convince me that Felix's inability to commit to dates meant he was married. He wasn't married.

There were so many times when we tried to meet; times I waited for him to tell me if he was free, if his work was done, if that conference call was over. So many times, I sent irritated messages and felt like a fool. I kidded him that his initials FTA meant Failure to Appear, a misdemeanor offense when a defendant didn't show up in court. Those initials became depressingly prophetic.

In one frustrated message to him, I parroted his opening line on CollarMe. "I thought we had that visceral connection you were looking for." I told him that I had feelings even if I was married, and I didn't like how I was being treated. I would later cringe at the *Fatal Attraction* cadence to my tone. I could almost see my face replacing Glenn Close's, flatly stating, "I will not be ignored," while incessantly clicking a table lamp off and on. I felt trapped in a cuckoo clock.

But I was not crazy. I was smitten. I was drowning in NRE and maybe even falling in love. We never got close enough for me to find out. Felix didn't let me in. I had not felt this way about anyone since I fell in love with Eric in college. I was scared and exhilarated at first; then, finally, lonely, humiliated, and depressed.

I would tell Eric that I might go out with Felix, whom he had never met, and then I would say, "Oh, never mind, he can't make it after all." It was a running joke, a heartbreaking one. I saw my husband with what I thought was pity in his eyes, or maybe it was sympathy, whenever I admitted to the latest instance of unfulfilled expectations. Feeling pitiful was not what I wanted from polyamory. It was hard for Eric to witness. My husband had a rough time with men he judged as disrespecting the woman he loved.

This emotional ping-pong lasted longer than it should have. Over the years—yes, years—I would see Felix maybe two or three times a year. Eventually, it petered out to even less. Every time, our connection was electric. Every time, I thought we would meet more often. Every time, he assured me he wanted that too, but something always intervened—his start-up business, primarily. Every time, after that first year, I initiated contact.

My sad sack reflection in the mirror derided me. *You're pathetic. This is what "He's not that into you" looks like. Stop reaching out.*

Something I read in the Dear Abby column when I was in middle school stuck with me. A wife wrote in about her cheating husband.

"What should I do—leave him or not?" she asked.

"Ask yourself the ultimate question," Abby replied. "Are you better off with him or without him? That's your answer."

"Better off" could mean emotionally, financially, physically, socially, or all of the above. Taking it all in, the good, the bad, the tolerable, would I rather be with him or be without him? When I thought about Felix, I realized that my pride was not that hard to swallow because I was not giving up anything except the time and effort to contact him, which, thanks to electrons, was minimal. The sweetness of the reward—our amazing connection—caused me to conclude that I was better off with him, even if I saw him only sporadically, rather than cutting him out of my life completely.

In the course of writing about my poly life, I talked with Felix. I was honest about how I felt about him and about the grand illusions I had when we first met. He admitted that he had felt the same strong connection but had been scared by its intensity and that he did not have full control over how it would play out because I was married.

"I don't get it. You were in a triad where you had two partners," I said.

"Yes, but I controlled all the points, not like with you."

"I think I was falling for you," I said.

"And I for you," he said.

I told him that I appreciated our talk. At a minimum, it made me feel less like I had imagined our relationship. We kept the door open for a time when his life was less hectic, and there could be an "us" in it. I suggested that he, Eric, and I have a drink together. He agreed.

"I think my experience with you caused me to pull back in later relationships," I told him.

"Same," he said.

"Meeting you was a turning point in my poly life," I said.

"How so?" he asked.

"You were the first guy I saw myself having a relationship with, not just an experience."

When he said he had felt the same way, my heart melted some, and the tension between my shoulders about us lessened. I doubted, however, that any future relationship would come of our chat, and I made peace with that.

I think Felix cared for me and wished we could have spent more time together, but wishing did not make it so, and I was not a wisher. I was a doer. I tired of prodding him with thirst-trap photos and invitations. It was humiliating. His relationship impotence finally crossed a line, transforming him from a mind-blowing connection worth fighting for, even if it only came to fruition as often as I correctly answered the Final Jeopardy Question, to a goddamn lost cause and a testament to my stubbornness at admitting failure.

Maybe one day, I'll see his name in the credits of an acclaimed film and think, yeah, I knew that guy; we had a moment. I would be genuinely happy for him.

I never figured out how to make a relationship work with someone who seemed to crave me with a panther-like hunger one minute and evaporate into the ether like a specter the next. I don't regret our relationship. It made me grow. It also made me doubt and overanalyze. For the duration, my circle of friends and my patient husband listened with empathy (predominantly) and affection (always). My many lifelines formed a safety net, so even when I felt I was falling off the poly ledge, I knew I never would. A dozen loving, interlocking hands would catch me and then hug me until I sobbed or laughed or screamed it all out—whatever I needed at the time. There was not a doubt in my mind.

* * *

After meeting Felix in my early poly exploration phase, I tried to figure out what kind of polyamory I was looking for. I didn't know yet what fit me. In the two months after Eric came home from Iraq and was dating Marianne, I had a few more dates with men from CollarMe because I already had the profile up.

There was the toppy surgical resident who worked long hospital hours. On our first date, we stopped at a CVS where he bought clothesline before we headed to the conveniently located ye olde Scotsman motel. He liked to create intricate Japanese-style shibari rope ties to decorate and restrain my body.

On a subsequent date, we met in a hotel room near his home, and he lashed my wrists over my head inside a doorway while I stood in five-inch stiletto heels and a thong for the hour it took for him to painstakingly complete the aesthetically beautiful knots. When I felt a tingling sensation in my wrists and my calf muscles complained, I asked for a break. He immediately unbound my wrists and carried me to the bed. I slid my thong down to my ankles and over my patent leather heels. He nestled his head between my thighs as I closed my eyes and enjoyed his unhurried attentions. He paused, and I inhaled, aroused. I waited for his next move. And waited.

I was about to say something when I noticed his breathing grow loud and steady. He was asleep. I laughed, but quietly. I slowly pulled my legs up under me, careful not to scrape my spiked heels on his neck.

I leaned over and gently shook his shoulder. "Hey," I whispered. "You fell asleep."

"Mm," he said behind closed eyes.

"I am going to go. You stay and rest. You need it."

I managed to move his sleepy form up the bed, so his head was on the pillow. I tucked the covers under his chin and left. He didn't fall asleep on our next date.

There was the lobbyist I met for afternoon coffee on our first date, and we walked to the hotel across the street for a spontaneous rendezvous. It was exciting to feel so desired by an attractive and interesting man that he could not wait to put his hands on me, and I was tantalized by the thought of how those hands—and mouth and tongue—would feel on me. He said he had a girlfriend who was cool with him dating. I insisted that he tell her of our impromptu outing, and he agreed. When he later decided not to tell her, I decided not to see him again.

There was also my Sex Delivery date, as I referred to him with Eric. I would drive to a single guy's place. He liked me to bring a sex toy that he would use on me. He handled the bullet-shaped, blood red vibrator with expertise, enjoying edging me gradually to ecstasy and then entering me and pounding me into the bed, his gold cross necklace dangling close to my face.

After sex, he talked of his search for the perfect girl to bring to Sunday dinners with his Catholic family. I would count the minutes before leaving without seeming like a dick. For a few years he would contact me occasionally to see if I wanted his attentions, as he called them. While the sex was hot, we had nothing else in common, so on balance, I thought not.

And there was the young, buff, gladiator-costumed blond I met dancing at a club on Halloween, a few months after Eric's return. I was Cleopatra in a white toga with black and gold edging, and I threaded gold beads through my dark brown bob. Eric was dressed as Antony in a sleeveless shirt and faux multi-paneled leather skirt that showed off his gym-muscled arms and legs. He won the prize for best costume. Eric offered to bring the gladiator home since, in his view, karma had brought him and Cleopatra together. I was excited at the prospect, so I asked him, and he said yes. We sat in the back seat while Eric drove with Marianne next to him.

At home, Eric and Marianne went to their usual upstairs bedroom, and the gladiator and I took the master bedroom. The gladiator's enthusiasm was invigorating and enduring, if manic and unfocused. I had to explain to him that anal sex was not first-date activity.

As we were relaxing after sex, he told me that he had been celebrating at the club because he had just turned twenty-one. My mouth gaped open and not to receive something good. For the only time in my life, I asked a guy if he had cab money to get back to his dorm.

The next morning over breakfast, Eric admired the ease with which I could hook up.

"Eric, I'm a chick. I'm relatively attractive, and I put out. It's not hard to find someone to shag me."

I, on the other hand, envied how he and his girlfriend asked about each other's day and texted heart emojis before saying good night. *Aww.* I wanted that too.

As I was discovering that finding an honest, lasting polyamorous relationship was not easy, I found myself considering something I never thought I would.

11.

Unethical Non-monogamy

The summer Eric was overseas and I was getting to know Felix, I started messaging with a man who lived in Chicago. We had immediate online chemistry. He traveled to the Washington area regularly for his work and had a hotel room when he did. We didn't spend much time discussing our home situations.

"Tell me a fantasy," he said.

"You may think it's passé, so don't laugh," I said, "but I have a fantasy of a silent stranger ripping off my clothes, buttons popping, because he can't wait to touch my bare skin."

He did not laugh. He told me in vivid detail how he would tempt and tease me, arouse me with his hands and tongue and take me to sensual places that lit me up from within. I was swept up in sexy chatting and exchanging provocative (but not fully nude) photos.

We finally addressed the logistics of what we had been working toward for several weeks. By this time, Eric had come home.

"I'm looking forward to finally meeting in person," I messaged.

"As am I," he responded. "The anticipation is excruciating."

His sometimes formal, almost stilted, tone of communicating added to my image of him as a dominant man who could help me explore the more sexually submissive dimension Felix had awoken. The fact that his profile name began with "Sir" only added to the mystique. When he betrayed his excitement at meeting me, I felt my need deepen.

"I know what you mean," I wrote. I visualized his lean, hard body from the bare-chested photos he had sent.

"Before we meet," I continued, "I need to know your full name and phone number. I give the information to my husband for safety. I'm sure you understand."

"I will give you what you request," he responded, "but I need to tell you that I am married. I am trusting your discretion. My wife does not know about this, and I don't want her to."

"Hold on," I wrote. "After weeks of talking and sending pictures, you are telling me this now?" I had been dying to act on our long-distance lustmance. I was not prepared to learn that he was married and planning to cheat on his wife.

"She finds my kinks distasteful and refuses to engage in them. I will certainly not force them on her." As far as I knew, he wasn't into anything violent or disgusting, but his wife had every right to choose not to participate.

"What about an open relationship? Have you talked about that?" Newbie poly me thought polyamory was the answer to everything. "You could get your needs met, and she wouldn't have to do what she didn't want to."

"She is not receptive to an open relationship," he said. "I have no plans to leave my wife or kids, so I arrange, infrequently, to seek out diversions." I assumed he and his wife still had sex, but I didn't ask.

All of this gave me pause, a lot of pause. I had not signed up to be the other woman. The whole idea was an uncomfortable reminder of my tenure as the cheated-upon wife.

"I don't like this. This is not how I engage," I told him. "I need to think."

"Okay," he responded.

The next day I messaged him. "I don't think it's a good idea for us to meet."

But . . . damn, I was spun up. I had invested time, energy, and salacious expectations. I could not stop myself from weighing the matter.

Cheating—to have intimate relations with someone not your partner without your partner's knowledge and consent—was *non*consensual non-monogamy and far from ideal, but it was certainly a reality. Men cheat. Women cheat. Nonbinary folks cheat.

If I slept with the Chicagoan, even though I was polyamorous and Eric knew about the meetup, it was still cheating because the married man's wife had not consented. Yes, you can still cheat if you are non-monogamous. If I did this, I would be a cheater, an adulterer, or an accomplice thereto. Since becoming polyamorous, Eric and I did not have sex with others without discussing it with each other and obtaining the informed consent of everyone involved.

How to deal with the question of cheating when it reared its throbbing head?

I wanted an erotic encounter that could lead to more encounters. That he had a hotel room when he came to town was so convenient for me. I didn't want to marry him or have his babies. I didn't want to disrupt his marriage or hurt his wife or family. I didn't live near them. I would never run into his wife.

I thought further. He had cheated before. And if not me, then it would be someone else.

Major rationalization. I knew it while I was doing it.

Then my psyche got vicious. Part of me thought she was selfish for denying him the opportunity to satisfy needs that she refused to meet. What was wrong with two adults—him and me—mutually satisfying each other? Who was *she* to stand in *our* way?

I was judging a woman I did not know, about her marriage, with my scale, weighted down with my longing to engage with her husband on all the levels we had been steamily discussing for two months.

My selfish rant ran away with me for a few minutes, and then I stopped and asked myself: Did I want to be *that* woman? Could I live with the notion that I had facilitated his adultery? And not just facilitated, but participated in.

My curiosity about what it would be like to be with him won out. He was as attractive in person as his photos showed, but more coldly distant than I had expected. Maybe it was part of his Dom persona. I was so new to kink that I had little idea.

We met at seven o'clock at a restaurant adjacent to his hotel. I was looking forward to getting an in-person vibe from him over dinner. And maybe a drink to settle my nerves.

After exchanging hellos, I looked at the menu. He did not.

"I've eaten," he said.

"I haven't," I said. Who meets at a restaurant at dinner time and doesn't eat?

"Feel free to order," he said. "You'll need your energy." His smile was so faint that I might have missed it if I had not been searching for a hint of reassurance in this encounter.

The restaurant was crowded and not conducive to intimate conversation. I ate my salad quickly, feeling his eyes on me.

He slid a key card across the table. "My room is 334. I will follow in five minutes. Disrobe and be ready for me."

How dominant. I was flushed with excitement. I wasn't sure exactly what would happen, but from our chat history, I had an idea it would be steamy.

As we were about to get down to it in the hotel room, the landline rang.

"I have to take this," he said.

He sat at the desk and answered the phone. His responses were concise and inflectionless, but I could tell it was his wife. If ever the universe was giving me a sign, there it was. I was an accomplice before the fact. I could still say, "I am not comfortable with this. I'm going to get dressed and go."

I walked to the bathroom, ostensibly to give him privacy, but even more to separate myself physically from the phone call and the situation. I looked in the mirror and parted my lips to form the words to say to him.

As I overheard one side of the married and mundane "how was your day?" conversation, I realized that I was irritated by her intrusion. It had been hard for me to enter the online dating world after being monogamous and married for years, and it was being made harder by the inconvenient reminder that he was married and cheating. We were cheating.

As he hung up, my ethical resolve wavered, then cratered. My curiosity, selfishness, and lust got the better of me. The thought of having a hot, local, no-strings, regular hookup was a wet dream I could actually live. I only had to silence the part of my brain that told me, *This is not right, and you know it.*

The tone of our ensuing sexual encounter should not have surprised me as soon as he told me not to make a mess because he frequented the hotel and did not want to telegraph his escapades. I felt filthy; not in a good, naughty, sexy way, but like a dirty secret, which of course I was.

Why did I go through with it? For once, I wanted to know what it felt like to be the other woman, to be the one who did not seem to care who her actions impacted, if anyone at all, and give in to recklessness, eroticism, and pure ego. I wanted to be selfish for a moment, like Katrina had been. Like Lorraine and Eric had been. Both women knew me. They knew Eric was married with a small child. I didn't know Chicago's wife, who lived half a dozen states away, and I never would.

And, pruriently, I wanted to know if the sexual experience would be as good as I had fantasized. It wasn't.

He messaged me the next time he was in town. I declined to meet him.

"Why did you go through with it before?"

"I was curious," I responded.

"What has changed?"

"I hate lying and cheating," I wrote, "and the sex was mediocre."

That was all true, but I did not say that about the sex. I said something like, "We were not as good a fit as I expected."

After I closed out the chat box on my phone, I wondered what I would have done if the sex had been of the can't-get-enough-or-I-will-die variety. Would I have swallowed the sourness of cheating, and if so, for how long?

Since that encounter, I have had to decide whether to engage with men who were not honest with their partners. In online exchanges, men told me that their marriages did not fulfill them sexually for a variety of reasons, including the mental and/or physical health of their partner and their unmet needs and proclivities. I cut communication off if they didn't have their partner's consent for their extramarital or extra-relationship activities. Some of them shouted me down for my declination, as in, "I am being up front about my situation. Isn't that what you women want? But I am being shut down for it anyway!"

I heard their frustration. I did. I was not unsympathetic to feeling trapped between love for a partner and a desire to explore outside the matrimonial bonds, especially if the marriage was a sexless one. I always suggested the man try honest dialogue with his wife about his wants, but I also understood that an open relationship model would not work for many—fear of asking, fear of being rejected, fear of being thought a pervert (like Chicago), and fear of losing one's marriage and kids. That all stemmed from the standard narrative that monogamy was the only valid relationship path and that any deviation therefrom was, well, deviant.

I learned to ask during our initial online exchange about the nature of my prospective date's arrangement with any partners. I found most men to be honest, and then it was up to me to decide. Some arrangements threw red flags in my way, such as a man's partner who was okay with him dating, but she did not want to date herself and did not want to know about it when he dated. That was a version of "Don't ask, don't tell."

DADT was a phrase reminiscent of the Clinton administration's problematic compromise policy of prohibiting discrimination against gays in the military, so long as they hid their sexual orientation and did not engage in homosexual acts. Forcing people to remain in the closet about who they were was itself discriminatory, and DADT was finally abandoned. In a polyamory context, DADT smacked of hypocrisy. Many polyamorists pushed back against it.

A DADT arrangement telegraphed to me that the girlfriend or wife was not on board but rather was tolerating his affairs for reasons that I was not privy to. The man's outside activities might technically have been condoned, but to me, it felt like cheating. I decided that I did not want to be part of DADT or cheating.

Eric had a brief dating relationship with a woman who was married with children and whose agreement with her husband was that she could date, but he did not want to know any details or meet anyone she dated. After the woman asked to be dropped off a block from her house after a date, Eric told me a DADT relationship was not for him. It felt sneaky and wrong. He had had enough of that kind of relationship.

On a first date with an online match, my date told me that he and his fiancée were trying to start a family and were house hunting, which were both stressful endeavors. She chose not to date and was pouty that he encouraged her to do so. She told him that his lack of jealousy at her dating meant he did not value her. Her response telegraphed to me that she had not accepted polyamory, and I stepped away from that potential land mine.

I met a man at a conference in Washington. We spent a lot of time together by virtue of our working relationship, and we hit it off, platonically. I could tell he was interested in me. I also knew he was married with small children, facts he did not hide. A flirty and extroverted sort, he hooked up with an unmarried mutual friend. Before their prearranged encounter, we were girl-chatting in her hotel room as she dressed for the date.

"Is he in an open marriage?" I asked.

"I assume not," she said. "I didn't ask."

I paused a beat. "Does that matter to you?"

"No," she said, pulling on her stockings. "I'm not in a position to evaluate their relationship, and it's not my job." She shrugged. "What he and I do is between him and me, here and now. What he chooses to tell his wife is up to him."

Soon after their affair, I was in his home city for work. I reached out to see if he wanted to save me from my distaste for solo dining. He jumped at the chance to rescue me and to show me a favorite restaurant overlooking the water. At dinner, I asked him if he was in an open marriage.

"No, I'm just a bastard," he said with a grin, his dimples deepening. "My wife and I have been together since high school. I'm the only lover she's had. I don't want her to regret not having more experiences. I tell her, 'Have a fling! Experiment,' but she won't."

I was uncomfortable with what he had revealed about his wife's sexual inexperience, so I didn't pry further. I did, however, tell him how it worked with me and Eric, whom he knew, and our dream of a world where non-monogamy was a normalized relationship choice. Well aware of how I had struggled with the concept and practice of polyamory, I tried not to judge others' relationship structures. I could only report what worked for me and hope that others might consider polyamory if their current relationship model wasn't meeting their needs.

I asked another polyamorist about his views on dating a married woman who was cheating. His view was like my gal pal's, with a locational caveat.

"I think I would be okay hooking up on occasion if, say, she was in town on business," he said. "That would put physical distance between me and her primary relationship."

"What if she was local?" I asked.

"No," he said. "I would feel uncomfortable pursuing a longer-term affair with a married woman who was local."

"Because of the likelihood of impacting her life and family?" I asked.

"Something like that," he said.

I respected him in many facets of his life, including being publicly transparent about his being polyamorous, so his response gave me pause. How would I react if the married and cheating guy was someone who made my pulse quicken? It was easy for me to wax virtuous when it mattered little.

A non-polyamorous friend in a D/s relationship repeatedly asked her Dom boyfriend if he was married, and he denied that he was, repeatedly. After falling in love with him, she found out he was married with children and cheating. When his wife found out, she was subpoenaed as a witness in an ugly divorce. She eventually extracted herself to move on to a healthier, honest relationship.

On my coastal work trip, my dimpled dinner companion and I never broached sex between us because, in the absence of consent from his wife, I was not on board. We finished our meal, and he walked me to my hotel. After a platonic hug, he went home to his family. We exchanged texts about how nice it had been getting to know each other better over seafood with a harbor view. I smiled at my phone and felt positive, if a little sexually frustrated.

12.
Permission

"Give yourself permission to be here," my massage therapist whispered.

At the start of our session, while I was face down and naked under a sheet, he told me to breathe deeply, exhale slowly, and relax. The muted lighting, lavender-scented oils, and lilting background music were designed to lull me, body and mind, to a place of calm.

As I breathed in and out, I willed the tension to flow from my core to the tips of my fingers and out into the universe. I tried to let go of the work week, the chores not done, the expectations I had for myself and for others. I tried to give myself permission to be myself and not to be anything to anyone else.

Tears flowed involuntarily from the corners of my eyes, dampening the sheet under my chin. I became quiet, embarrassed at my emotional breakdown. What was wrong with me?

That my masseur started the session by asking me to allow myself to be selfish for a little while and to let someone tend to me conveyed that it was not unusual for his clients to need that reminder. I felt like a cliché of an uptight professional who couldn't unclench herself long enough for the hippy-dippy tracks on the CD to play out.

Massage was intimate. I was vulnerable, naked. I was at the tender mercies of an almost stranger, whose hands touched my flesh, kneaded my aches, and held my pain.

Once his ask was articulated, the question of whether I could permit myself to be selfish for an hour took on physical mass, pressing on my temples, reminding me of everything that waited for me when I left the cocoon of his studio. I could not relax. I stopped getting massages. The experience was too raw.

I fumed to myself, *I do not need to pay good money to feel uncomfortable and blubber on a folding table. This is supposed to be relaxing. I feel like I should be in a caftan with wands of incense being waved over me so that the negative energy can be exorcised from my aura, or whatever.*

But I had to ask myself why complying with his seemingly simple directive was so hard.

With the opening of my marriage to dating separate partners, I sometimes felt like giggling, goggled Minions were crashing bumper cars against my insides.

If it was that hard to allow myself fifty minutes of therapeutic touch a few times a year, how could I give myself permission to embrace a polyamorous life every day?

My worries about being selfish in tending to my emotional and physical desires seemed unfounded when I saw the relative ease with which my husband immersed himself in polyamory. Eric did not change who he was by being polyamorous. He did not abandon the other aspects of his nature and his life, except for monogamy. He supplemented them.

Perhaps I was the victim of working-mom guilt and the fear that my emotional life was a zero-sum equation. Time is finite, but our capacity to love and care for one another is not. A central tenet of polyamory refutes the cultural narrative that we can only truly love one person romantically at a time by asserting that our ability to form multiple intimate connections simultaneously is limited only by the time we can devote to the relationships.

Choosing a polyamorous life or recognizing and accepting that I was polyamorous was permission I wanted to give myself. Why did I feel guilty?

I didn't feel guilty for caring for someone outside of my marriage. I felt guilty that I was shirking responsibilities in favor of irresponsibility and, dare I say it, fun. I thought that *fun* was a dirty word that serious-minded wives and mothers—monogamous, faithful people—were not supposed to spend precious time on unless that fun included a child or spouse, ideally both.

Before I left for a date, I might do a load of laundry or be sure there was food for dinner for Eric and Will in the fridge. I did the same before I traveled out of town for work. I ticked the box labeled "Family/Work/House Taken Care Of" before I considered the box that said "Natalie Taken Care Of."

Eric rolled his eyes mightily at my box-checking. "Natalie, go, have fun. Then come home so I can see in your eyes, and hear in your voice, that you did. That will make me smile. We can take care of ourselves here."

Maybe it was not guilt but fear that how I defined a large part of me was not all of me; that who I was included being polyamorous, being someone else's lover or girlfriend or metamour; that after so many years of being a monogamous momwife, my identity had shifted. My psyche needed time to catch up.

I operated best within structures, so I developed a ritual. It helped me grant myself the grace to be fully polyamorous—someone other than a housewife, mother, or wage-earner. I could be a lover, a girlfriend, a sexual being, a karaoke queen, or whatever else polyamory meant for me.

After I dolled myself up, gathered my bag of tricks, and GPS'd my route (and, okay, folded the laundry), I told Eric I was on my way out and what time I expected to be home. I looked into his warm brown eyes, smiled, told him I loved him—because I did, and do, so very much—and bounded out the door, full of joy at the permission I had given myself to explore new connections, and even to have fun.

13.
Getting Real

Marianne was a smart, scrub-faced, ponytailed Midwesterner pursuing graduate studies at Georgetown University. She and Eric met within a month of his return from Iraq. Although younger than Eric by twenty years, she was more experienced at polyamory. Both of her prior long-term relationships had been polyamorous. In one, she was the primary partner, and in another, she was the secondary. She seemed to wear polyamory as naturally as goth girls wore black.

Marianne, Eric, and I practiced a form of *hierarchical polyamory*, where we accepted that Eric and Marianne's relationship was secondary to Eric's relationship with me by virtue of the ties that bound us in a long-term intimate marriage, parenthood, joint bank accounts, and shared history and responsibilities. If Eric were forced to choose between us, he would choose me. As a result, I did not feel threatened that she wanted Eric for a monogamous relationship where I was baggage to be jettisoned. My relief was momentous after the agony and uncertainty of Lorraine.

In our every interaction, I could see that Marianne respected our marriage. She seemed to derive nourishment from being part of our freaky family. Marianne regularly spent weekends at our house, away from her roommate, who didn't approve of polyamory or Marianne and Eric's generational age gap. She would help Eric assemble a weight bench or an Ikea bookcase on a "chore date," as Eric called them. She might borrow our car to run errands. She and Eric might talk about her graduate school courses and career prospects in public policy, as that was the focus of Eric's military role. On a few occasions, she used our well-equipped kitchen to cook meals, leaving some for us, before packing the bulk to take back to her small apartment.

Marianne would join Eric, Will, and me for dinner when she stayed overnight. Will didn't know about our non-monogamous life, but he was used to having our friends at the house, as well as having them sleep over. Ever since Helen came to live with us after I broke my arm, when Will was ten, the presence of other adults, especially women, was normal. Will had an ease with adults that I think came from being an only child. Since he was a toddler, Will was exposed to Eric's conviviality and our cadre of friends.

During the blossoming of our post-swinging poly life, Will was an adolescent. He knew what sex was, but we did not talk to him about what we did behind closed doors. I reasoned that no kid wanted to think about their parents' sex lives with each other, much less with other people.

Maybe we should have been more evolved, and maybe I was old-fashioned and unenlightened in this regard, but frankly, my sex life was none of my son's business. It was a private adult matter. And, knowing Will—who said he was "scarred for life" after his fourth-grade health class about sex—talking to him about polyamory would be as welcome as ants at a picnic.

I hear you saying *but Natalie, poly is not all about sex*. Yes, yes, true. It's not *all* about sex. It's about emotional intimacy and all the aspects of a relationship.

But it is also about sex. Any serious discussion about polyamory and dating cannot ignore the physical aspect. No, Will's head would not have spun around like an *Exorcist* remake if we had told him about polyamory. However, this was the same kid who said he needed comfort food when I revealed I had my navel pierced while on vacation with Eric in Ibiza, after he asked not only if I was having a midlife crisis and whether Dad knew (yes, he was with me), but called my piercing The Abomination. Hefty verbiage coming from a middle schooler. I tried not to laugh too hard in his cute face. But I digress.

Yet only slightly because I thought what we told Will was an individualized decision that depended on our particular child, not on a script, not on what a book advised, and not what other polyamorous parents did. What to tell Will about the poly part of our lives was a considered decision. I feared it was the kind of reveal that could fund a therapist's Malibu beach house.

Eric was in a relationship with Marianne, and he wanted to come clean, especially since Marianne was regularly at our house. Will knew that she stayed over, and while he may have wondered why, he never asked or seemed concerned. We have had adult, platonic housemates over the years, starting with Helen. When a barber politely asked ten-year-old Will if he had any siblings, my only child said without pausing, "Yes, a sister. She's twenty-eight," referring to Helen.

If something did not directly concern him, Will didn't ask about it. More than once, I was traveling for work, and he would ask Eric, "What time is Mom coming home?" Eric would remind him that I was out of town, had been for two days, and would be back tomorrow. "Oh, okay," he would say.

"Why do you want to tell him we date?" I asked Eric. "Because it would be easier for you? Because you don't like lying to him, and you think that's what we're doing?"

"Yes, mainly," he said.

I, too, worried that Will might resent our dishonesty, but I foresaw the downside of burdening and potentially hurting my child with something he wasn't ready to hear. I asked Eric to put himself in Will's place. Would you want to know that your parents were screwing others? Wouldn't that shake your secure little world? Wouldn't you wonder if anyone your parents talked to was a fuck buddy and picture them screwing all their friends in your home? *Ew.*

I considered using our relationship as a teaching model and saying to Will, "Hey, kiddo, we love and respect each other, and this is our choice." I did not choose that path. I didn't want to risk adding to our son's struggles. Middle school was rough enough. Was I overprotective, ill-informed, or just a coward? Possibly one or more. Feel free to judge. I knew one couple who told their son, and that knowledge made him doubt his parents' relationship. I knew parents whose kids knew their mom's boyfriend as a close family friend. That was our typical model with Will.

Eric and I agreed that if Will asked, we would not lie to him because his asking would mean he was ready. We would deal with the potential blowback of "Wait, what? So, that friend of Dad's who slept over was his girlfriend? And that friend of Mom's who lent me a stack of comics—you were sleeping with him?

How could I be so stupid? I wonder if my friends suspect. Who else knows? Aunt Jessie? The Millers? Am I the last one?"

If this sounds like we were hiding from our son, we were. At that time, we were concealing our lifestyle from our jobs, our neighbors, and many of our friends and family members. Even my former therapist didn't understand, much less accept my polyamory as anything but aberrant.

Were we being false by not broadcasting our relationship dynamic? Did we owe the world an explanation? Those were loaded questions. Over the course of my polyamorous life, I struggled with some of them daily, but Eric and I found a workable middle ground. That ground shifted, but it didn't crack wide open and swallow us whole. The longer we were polyamorous, the more comfortable we became sharing that fact, and the wider our circle of friends and relatives, and even employers, who learned about that aspect of our lives.

Eric and I have been in public with our other partners. Perhaps we were observed holding hands, leaning in across a restaurant table, or kissing on a street corner. If so, no one has commented to either of us. No one told either of us, "I saw your spouse with someone else, and I thought you should know. They were coming out of a hotel/kissing/gazing into each other's eyes." Perhaps most people suspected my marriage was not a traditional one. When someone asked me, I didn't lie to them. Over time, I became less concerned about what other people thought of how I lived my life now, but that was not always so.

Like many parents, I hid things from my child. I didn't tell him that while he was at school, the cancer-ridden family dog visited the vet a final time. I told him our pet had died at home. When he was in kindergarten and asked where babies came from, I didn't explain penis-in-vagina intercourse. I gave him an age-appropriate answer. In this life, there is enough hurt, change, disruption, and confusion that we cannot protect our kids from. I assumed he would either figure it out or ask sooner or later. That turned out to be later.

One weekend afternoon, Marianne was wrestling with Will on the carpet. At thirteen, Will had a couple of inches on Marianne, but she was powerful and fit. I envied her muscled legs and her ability to bench-press her weight. They got along in an easy familial way. She reminded him, "Will, take your plate to the kitchen," and asked him which belt he was up to in martial arts. It was no secret that Marianne wanted to start a family someday. Eric grinned and told her, "I look forward to dancing at your wedding and spoiling your children."

Despite Marianne's small footprint and pleasant manner, having my husband's lover in my home space so often was challenging. My discomfort was not with Marianne as an individual, but with how Eric's poly relationship preferences were different than mine. Eric liked to integrate his lovers into our life. He liked to have breakfast with his lover on one side and his wife on the other. His way was called *kitchen table polyamory*, meaning that members of the polycule were friendly and integrated enough to eat a meal together. Our group interactions served as tangible confirmation to him that polyamory was working.

As for me, my lovers rarely slept over and stayed for breakfast. They did not hang out on weekends or cook meals at our house like Eric's girlfriends did. They didn't pick up our mail or water our plants when we were away. Was that because my partners were men? Was it because most were married, and my husband's lovers were single? Maybe a bit of all of that.

I didn't think I wanted what Eric wanted. I didn't need my lovers to share meals and be part of the household. I already had a family, and the guys I dated were not interested in that. I told myself that I was not looking for a second spouse, or even a sometimes lover to make regular appearances in my home. During the time Eric was dating Marianne, I usually met my dates outside the house, savoring the freedom to explore who I was away from my identities as wife and mother.

Even though I didn't want the integration of my lovers into my homelife, I sometimes felt stung by Eric and Marianne's relationship—affectionate and comfortable, even domestic. When I would walk in on them at the house, her sitting on his lap in our shared office while they laughed at something online or he offered mentoring advice, I felt as if I were intruding. Eric would smile and tell me I was not, with a "Hi, Natalie, what's up?" or "Come sit with us." I believed him, but in those moments, I felt the weighty absence of affection and familiarity from my dating life. For the first few months of their relationship, I was seeing a couple of men casually, but I did not have the loving connection that Marianne and Eric had.

Marianne's presence in the house impacted me in unpredictable ways. I could get testy with her, which made me feel like a bad polyamorist. It was psychological work for me to have her at the house. She wasn't a guest, and she wasn't a family member. She was something in between, for which there was no Miss Manners to consult.

"Hey, Nat, Eric said to put the sheets and towels on top of the washer. Is that okay? I am happy to wash them myself." I knew she would have cheerfully done whatever I asked within reason.

"No, it's fine," I said, "I have to do the rest of the laundry anyway."

I bristled a little at being the laundress for the mistress, but it seemed petty to ask her or him to do them. Laundry had always been my chore in our marital division of labor. I liked the order of dirty in and clean out. It was not the soiled sheets that bothered me as much as my envy of Eric living a charmed life with his wife and girlfriend nestled in his home, whereas I was still looking for Mr. Polyamorous. I felt pathetic, like being picked last for fourth-grade kickball, and that made me irritable. Eric liked offering Marianne a refuge from her small apartment, whereas I would have preferred they stay at her place more often. He liked having her as part of the family.

I wanted to grow into a more generous person. I really did. But polyamory felt like drawing the short straw. I rationalized that it was good for me to open my home as well as my heart to Eric's lovers, but I also wanted space. My husband's girlfriend camped out on the sofa, working on her laptop while I did laundry, ran errands, or cooked meals for the week. I could not help but wonder how Eric would feel if my lovers spent so much time at the house. Then I had to admit that Eric most likely would have been more welcoming than me, but he was not tested in those early days.

I tried to be friendly. I attempted to talk to Marianne about my other relationships, but she seemed reluctant to engage. Maybe that was because she hesitated to say anything that might upset me.

About four months after Eric and Marianne started dating, my new boyfriend was navigating our dating and his marriage. Sometimes, for no reason apparent to me, he would tell me that he felt he should stay in with his wife rather than go out with me, despite the absence of a request from his wife. I got the impression he felt his volunteering to be with her would earn him good husband points, even though his wife, who had a boyfriend, bristled visibly and audibly at any perceived manipulation of her emotions.

Marianne and Eric were in our kitchen when I got my boyfriend's text canceling our weekly date.

"He told me, 'I am just trying to keep everyone happy.'" I grumbled. "Well, *I'm* not happy. Doesn't that matter?"

Eric said, "Give the guy a break; he's doing his best."

I rolled my eyes.

Marianne was silent, even though I would have welcomed her perspective.

A few days later, she told me, "Natalie, it's hard for me to hear you complain about your lack of time with your boyfriend. I cherish each moment with Eric. I am grateful for any time we have."

While I understood Marianne's point of view, her comments made me feel like a whiner. What was vastly different in our situations, in my view, was that she saw Eric at least twice as often as I saw my other partner. I was more generous in sharing my time and home space than was my other metamour, who was incredulous that I permitted Marianne in *my* house so often, much less let her stay overnight.

"I would not put up with it," she said to me. "You are the wife."

"It's Eric's home, too," I told her. "It's a big house. I am trying to be hospitable. We are poly. We make room for partners."

"I'm the queen bee in my house. End of story."

That explains a lot, I thought.

Typically, I slept alone when Eric had Marianne or occasionally another lover in the spare room. He made a point of checking in with me the morning after with a smile and a kiss, which I appreciated. He and Marianne would make breakfast when she stayed over, and we would eat together if I was not running to the gym for a weekend class.

That morning tranquility was not always easy to achieve, but I worked at it, and Marianne was unfailingly pleasant and accommodating, surely sensing my discomfort at feeling like the third wheel at my own breakfast table. Nonetheless, unkindness could spill out of me if not deliberately checked. Tangible evidence of their more fulsome relationship, such as condom packets in the trash can or a spanking paddle on the garage workbench, rankled me.

Marianne dated other men, but she did not have another serious relationship during the three years she was my metamour. Eric, however, dated other women while he was seeing Marianne. Gracie, for instance, was a stealth metamour. Her impact on me was negligible. She was single and saw Eric monthly or quarterly, depending on whether she was pursuing a monogamous relationship with someone else. I had met Gracie a few times, including dinner at our house. While we had a spare key to her apartment in case of emergency, when it came to *metamour maintenance*—yes, we coined a word for it—she needed almost none.

Marianne ended her romantic relationship with Eric to pursue monogamy with a guy who would not consent to her seeing Eric. His refusal was heartbreaking to both Marianne and Eric. Having no familiarity with and even less tolerance for polyamory, the new guy was wary of starting a relationship with her while Eric was still in the picture.

Marianne was a wonderful metamour. It was not her fault that I was still growing into my polyamorous life, still far from where I wanted to be. I was in the early stages of navigating being a secondary to my new boyfriend's wife, cataloging Lorraine's offenses and vowing to eschew them. I had hoped that Marianne would be a convenient resource for me as I embarked on my secondary status since she was experienced in that role. However, my expectations were unfair to Marianne. Although she answered some of my poly questions, I often noticed her reticence when I asked for advice.

Marianne understood relationship boundaries but was not afraid to ask Eric for what she wanted. That might be a night out to the kink club, a trip to the beach, or more time alone together. I tried to respect Marianne's requests and talked with Eric when they were at odds with mine. It was an effort for me to be smiley and supportive about yet another overnight trip when I did not have the same luxury with my lovers. I saw in hindsight that she might have wondered where my boundaries were, as they could shift with my mood.

While we were far apart in age (Millennial and Gen Xer), worked in different industries (policy wonk versus trial lawyer), and spent our leisure time in dissimilar ways (she liked Ultimate Frisbee and running; I liked solo gym time and core classes), I was aware that Marianne had my back; whether she knew it, I also had hers.

She might not have known that when Eric was conflicted, frustrated, or even fatalistic about their relationship and its trajectory, given her expectations—was it possible for him to fulfill her wants and needs when he was a busy, married, working, co-parent?—I offered him perspective.

"Eric, perhaps you should talk to her about how you feel, rather than unilaterally deciding to break up. Marianne is a bright, rational woman. I know you love her. Why not tell her what's on your mind and listen to her response?"

"We'll see," he would say noncommittally.

That happened more than once.

And more than once, he came home not having broken up. I was glad of that. Even with my periodic discomforts, I liked Marianne, and I liked that their relationship brought him far more happiness than turmoil.

Because of the integration of Marianne into our lives, she was privy to familial goings-on as we discussed our son, financial matters, or the health of aging parents. She was not intrusive and maintained a balance that often awed me. It made me love Eric even more that he had chosen an emotionally intelligent woman to love and cherish.

While Eric was dating Marianne and I had a boyfriend, my father lived in our guest room so I could take him to oncology appointments. I thought more than once about telling Dad about my poly life, but he was sick, and Marianne came around much less while Dad was in the room she would have occupied. I was fairly certain that Dad would have said something like, "I just want you to be happy." Even so, I didn't want to burden him with information that didn't seem necessary, especially when he was engaged in what would be a losing battle with cancer.

Three months later, when Eric, Will, and I returned from Dad's out-of-town funeral, I could swear the kitchen smelled of food. Had I left something out? Looking around, I saw no evidence of it. I chalked it up to my fatigue and went to bed.

The next morning, I opened the fridge. A neatly covered Pyrex baking dish sat on the shelf. I could not remember it being in there or what it was. *How tired am I that I don't remember this? I do all the household cooking.*

I lifted the corner of the foil to discover Marianne's signature Tater Tot Hot Dish, a casserole that Will adored. My throat tightened and my eyes misted. I texted her immediately.

"Thank you, kitchen elf, for the delicious surprise. You are a treasure. ♥ Natalie."

After their amicable if emotional breakup, Marianne remained part of Eric's life, and thus mine. I generally knew what was going on with her, through Eric, social media, and our occasional texts or check-ins with each other. I could not know exactly how Marianne and Eric's relationship would morph, but I sensed she would remain in our lives. Their genuine expressions of love via text or phone were an example to me of how polyamory could be, at least one version of it. That was a version I sometimes was wistful for. I had hoped that their tender and mutually supportive dynamic was one I could strive for when I became a secondary.

Then, at long last, came my first real polyamorous relationship.

14.
Here Comes a Relationship

The more I saw Eric and Marianne's relationship grow, the more dissatisfied I became with the casualness of dating single guys who were not polyamorous. The turning point might have come after the surgical resident who fell asleep between my legs gave me the "it's not you, it's me" speech when he wanted to rekindle a relationship with an old flame who had dumped him for someone who had, in turn, ditched her. I wished him well and moved on.

Like a Colorado miner sifting through mountains of silt, I examined online profiles in search of a gold nugget. I was bemoaning aloud my latest dating failure when Eric suggested I try the OkCupid dating site—OKC for short—where he had met Marianne. I made a profile and filled an hour in a mammogram waiting room answering hundreds of questions for an algorithm to ingest and spit forth my perfect matches. I later realized I should have kept some answers private, based on the prurient responses I received. Being honest about how often I preferred sex and what turned me on was a siren song to the unwashed masses, some of them literally.

"Hey, baby, I know what you like, you dirty bird. My big dick will rock your world. I can send you a photo if you give me your email address or phone number." Reading my inbox made me grimace as if I had stepped in manure.

The few photos I posted on my dating profile obscured my face out of concern for being recognized by colleagues on the same site. The sexual aspect of polyamory constituted the crime of adultery where I lived, making being polyamorous technically illegal. Not a great look for someone who enforced the law. I had to be careful. My profile pictures showed me wearing sunglasses or with my hair in my face. In one picture, I was dancing with my midriff revealed and my hair falling across my face. In another, I used a picture from a photoshoot where I was reclining on a desk. I cropped the photo from the nose up to hide my face, but reveal my smile, the swing of my bobbed hair, sheer stockings and shiny stilettos.

The photos telegraphed sexuality, but my summary was excruciatingly detailed. Anyone who looked past the provocative pictures would read in the first paragraph that I was ethically non-monogamous because I wrote: "I am polyamorous. I am married to a great guy. I am looking for dating relationships and local adventures."

Per the site's prompts, I listed the bands, movies, books, and food that I liked. I attempted to describe my ideal guy without sounding pretentious or shallow. Try that as a writing prompt.

I said, "Wit, physique, and intelligence matter to me, so share a photo that shows more than your wicked smile, although that counts for a lot. I posted mine, so fair is fair." I was not interested in someone who defined themselves solely by the sports team they followed or their political party, any party. I mentioned I was in a book club, liked dancing in the wee hours to VNV Nation, and made a mean gumbo. Borrowing from Felix, I concluded with a request for those who were looking for a visceral connection.

I received messages immediately. My first date was with a wheat-haired guy in his early thirties who told me that he was familiar with polyamory. We met on a weekday evening. The Chinatown bar he chose was crowded, and we had to hustle our way into the bartender's line of sight. She asked for our IDs. I grudgingly handed over my driver's license as if parting with a C-note, watching closely for any reaction. I was more than ten years older than my date. She remained expressionless.

We sat at a high top and sipped our drinks. We chatted easily. I liked his smile. The bar was noisy, so after we finished our drinks, we walked outside.

"I'm very attracted to you," he said.

I was flattered. "Thank you."

"I want to take you to my place," he said, fixing his eyes on mine.

I was tempted but said, "I don't think so, but thanks."

"Maybe another time." He smiled, and we parted ways. I never heard from him again.

I was attracted to him, but I did not want a hookup. I wanted something else, something more. I wasn't sure what it was, but to paraphrase Justice Stewart, I figured I'd know it when I saw it.

* * *

Two weeks into my online dating presence, I was in my office during the quiet week between Christmas and New Year's Day. I checked the OKC phone app for messages and saw I had a new one:*

> Well, I'm not some bloody gym rat, but I keep in good shape. I can ride down most any fool on my bike. That's about all I'm willing to say regarding my "physique." I'd rather connect based on personality, and no, that does not mean I'm some fucking landwhale. Other than that, I was wondering what club that was in your second picture. I thought I'd been to most of the decent joints in the city, but, if it's goth night, and I've missed it, I need to get on that.
>
> But yeah, hi, I'm Hank. I'm completely bloody insane, and I like loud music. Also, the concept of a book club that doesn't read garbage like *Tuesdays With Morrie*, or *The Da Vinci Code*, or *The Girl With The Dragon Tattoo* (which, sadly, I did read on vacation some years back, and realized was worse self-insert fanfiction than *Twilight*) is damned intriguing. But yeah. Cool. I dunno.

Apparently, even more bored than I was when I signed up for the site, Hank had answered over five hundred questions. Our algorithm match was 95 percent. He was cute, with short, almost black hair and an aquiline nose. In only one picture did he smile. It was a nice smile. I later discovered that he cropped someone out of that photo—his mom. Hence the pleasant smile.

---

* The quoted exchanges with Hank are substantially verbatim, edited for brevity.

I also later learned that the photo was more than ten years old and showed a Hank at least twenty pounds lighter, but hey, that's all part of online dating. There is typically some bait and switch going on. I, for instance, listed my age as five years younger than I was. May I please blame being raised on *Seventeen* and *Cosmopolitan* and impossible ideals for women? Okay, maybe that's a cop-out. I paid for that lie later. Assuming Hank's reported age of thirty was true, I was fifteen years older than him.

His other dating site photos included him sticking his stud-pierced tongue out to a cartoonish length, flashing the devil's horns sign with his index finger and pinky, and brows knitted while working on a computer repair.

I read his summary page and his answers to many of the half-a-thousand questions. He was married and polyamorous, like me. His wife, Sylvia, was eight years his senior per her dating profile, which he had linked to his. She had commented on his profile page, presumably to show he was not cheating on her.

In the category of things he could not do without, Hank listed his leather jacket, music, books, his dog, his wife, and either horror movies or comics, I can't recall. I admired the punch of his message, his way with words, and his irreverence. He sounded fun and a little dangerous.

From behind my desk, which faced my office door, my computer screen hiding my face, I bent over my phone and tapped out a response:

> Okay, you got my attention. I'm a bit intrigued / exhausted by your ADHD summary and photos. I love that your wife wrote on your summary. Cool. Really cool. That picture is from the Crypt. The deejays play a lot of goth industrial and some '80s (my weakness).
>
> So, yep, I admit that I'm shallow regarding appearances when it comes to dating... okay... fucking. Sorry, them's the facts. That's why the photo requirement.
>
> I dunno either.

We continued in that vein, trading a couple dozen messages during the workday.

Hank responded, "Aren't we all shallow? I suppose I'm not one to pass said physicality test. Le fucking sigh."

I shot back, "I showed you a picture of me, so it's not like I'm being unfair, but your call. If you see me at the Crypt, be sure to tell me I'm a vain bitch, pull up your shirt to tease me, and then dance that crazy stompy way I bet you dance."

"Did the death metal and leather jacket give it away?" he asked.

I rolled my eyes and laughed. "Call me psychic, but I just don't see you two-stepping to metal."

He continued, "As for dancing, I should prepare my finest tuxedo and waltzing shoes. I would need a proper cane, not some ridiculous steampunk thing, and hat. Damn these ideas that take haberdashers to implement!"

I replied, "You win. I don't think I have seen anyone use haberdasher in context in, well, ever."

Hank said, "I think I need some chips to get back in this game, I'll take lighthearted discussion for 400, Alex."

Trying to dismount the verbal roller coaster, I asked, "How about I buy you a drink instead?" No one could be this zany in real life.

"Sure, we can totally do that. Wherever's clever."

I was looking forward to meeting the proprietor of this witty wordplay. During our online banter, Hank told me his wife's boyfriend played Legos with her son/his stepson and attended family events like the annual Zombie Walk.

That is so great! I thought. *That's how Marianne is with us. His wife Sylvia has a long-term boyfriend, so she must be cool with poly and with Hank dating. Plus, she is experienced at poly, and that will make this all easier.*

I learned that Sylvia's son and mine were born just a few weeks apart. Sylvia's dating profile impressed me as self-assured, direct about what she wanted, and genuine—if a bit snarky. We were two poly and married working moms. I was jazzed at the possibilities of being a secondary to a married poly guy with a wife not so different from me and my chance to be The Best Secondary I Could Be!

Hank and I agreed to meet at four o'clock the next day, since the holiday week meant early outs from work. When I caught sight of Hank, he was leaning against a street sign, wearing a leather jacket over a black T-shirt and black jeans, looking like he "was about to rob someone"—his words. He was fiddling with his phone and scowling a bit.

I was in work clothes that could double as date clothes during a nearly empty office week—an above-the-knee black skirt, form-fitting beige sweater, black trench coat, and calf-high boots. I had worn stockings that looked like watercolor tattoos of six-inch goldfish swimming up my legs.

We walked to the dive bar I had chosen in my attempt to telegraph an easy coolness, only to discover that it was not open yet. To kill time, we strolled a loop of a few city blocks at a brisk pace in the cold. Making first-date small talk while walking meant mainly looking straight ahead or else risk running into a parking meter or office escapees before the long weekend.

We talked about holiday traditions. For his family of three, he had served a Christmas duck. I was impressed. I did not know anyone who cooked duck, especially anyone wearing a black shirt broadcasting in white Courier type, YOUR DAUGHTER IS TIED UP IN A BASEMENT IN BROOKLYN. He also told me of his default disdain for most lawyers, his bosses in particular. The universe was a pistol, I thought.

After our second pass of the bar, we ventured down the dark interior steps and found it open. We slid onto barstools, and Hank quizzed the barkeep about the choices for cheap whiskey.

Our conversation at the bar was a trade-off of jibes, snipes, and smart-ass remarks as if we were in middle school, acting as if we didn't even like each other and our friends had set us up, or something. It was not unlike our online chat of the day before, and it was unlike any date I'd ever had.

Hank volunteered that he had been arrested more than once, including the time he had face-punched a Scientologist on the street for a "good reason." He had done most drugs, including smoking pot daily since middle school. He once dyed his hair green and showed me an old driver's license to prove it. He had been sexually active from an age that made me flinch. He chain-read books on his phone, most of which he stole via tech sorcery I did not grasp.

"I'm only good at two things," he told me, absent emotion. "Sex is one of them."

"Noted," I said. "And the other?"

"I know where to eat. I've lived here most of my life."

I sensed he was also good at his computer tech job. Why did I think that? Oh, yes, I remember—because he told me. Did this guy have a huge ego or just no filter because why bother?

We sat side-by-side on bar stools, still not facing each other. His monologue stunned me into silence. While Hank downed shots of rail whiskey, I sipped a lager. Gazing into my pint glass as if it held answers, I tried to think of what to say.

My cocksure online banter seemed like a ruse now. I had never been arrested, not even close. The one time I skipped school in ninth grade with a friend, we didn't have the sense to call the school and give an excuse, so they contacted my mother at work, and we were immediately busted. I colored inside the lines. Hank struck me as someone who smashed crayons with his fist, smeared the garbled colors on paper, and wrote expletives over the page in black marker.

I had never punched anyone beyond some grade school tussling with a pug-shaped, cul-de-sac bully with a bowl haircut named Joey Canestri. And drugs? No competition there. I wondered what he saw in boring, inexperienced me. I asked myself what I was getting into with someone who might be a helluva lot more—more of what I was not sure—than I had bargained for.

There seemed to be no end to his stories, including going to Georgetown for his first tattoo. He called it Death on a Shitter. I raised an eyebrow.

"I asked for the cheapest tattoo they had. The guy pointed to one, and I said 'sure.'" He pulled up his pant leg, and inked on his calf was a skeleton sitting on a toilet. Hank tossed back another shot and excused himself.

I checked my phone. Eric had texted.

Eric: How's the date? Do you think you'll be coming back here?

Me: He's outside smoking.

Eric: Ugh.

Me: Yeah.

Eric: Well, good luck. Marianne and I will be in the upstairs guest room. You guys can have the master if you end up here.

Me: Not likely, but thanks.

Eric: Love you.

Me: Ditto.

The winter sky was darkening when Hank returned from his smoke. He asked what I wanted to do next. I wavered. I did not see the date going anywhere, but it was early, and Eric and Marianne would be occupied literally over my head at home. I figured, well, he's amusing, and I don't have a better plan. What the hell.

On the twenty-minute cab ride from the Chinatown bar to the particular watering hole he favored in Adams Morgan, Hank regaled me with more anecdotes. Ten minutes into a first date, his date's boyfriend showed up unexpectedly—at least unexpectedly to Hank, who took his leave. "Hell, it's not that I mind meeting your boyfriend, but give a guy some warning," he told her.

We drank more. Hank drank much more than me because I am a lightweight, and I estimated he had eighty pounds on me. There was a no-bullshit way about him. He told me things about himself and his childhood on a first date that I wouldn't reveal on the tenth, vulnerable things, real things that are too personal for me to repeat. Somehow, this world-weary, thirty-year-old with gnawed fingernails was growing on me.

We were the only customers in a dim, dank upstairs bar that looked like a ship's hull after a fire. I noticed that Hank engaged the bartenders in each place we went, projecting that he was happy to be in their establishment and wanted them to have a good evening, asking, "Hey, how ya doing?" In an age of credit card transactions, he always had cash for the tip jar.

We took our five-buck beers to a table that looked like it had been built from driftwood a century ago. I propped up my feet on the bench next to Hank as we faced each other across the table. My feet were tired from the kitten-heeled suede boots I had been wearing all day. He casually rested his hand on my calf.

Our afternoon date had involved several blocks of walking, a cab ride, and had landed us at three different bars. Lunch had been nine hours ago, and I was feeling the four beers sloshing in my empty stomach. I set my drained pint glass down.

"I've got to eat something," I said. "Are you hungry?"

"I ate at home before I met up with you, but, sure, there's a decent pizza joint nearby," Hank said. "Do you like pizza?"

"I do indeed like pizza."

I managed, barely, to make it down the rowhouse bar's narrow winding staircase. Bracing my palms against the cool, stone walls helped steady me. The street was alive with pedestrians, traffic noises, and televisions blaring from sports bars below street level. The pizza place, a block down, was brightly lit. I ordered a long slice.

"If you want a bite," I said, "you better speak up now."

"Nope. Do you." Hank watched as I folded the cheesy triangle in half on the thin paper plate and inhaled it.

"Better," I said.

"What, no burp?" Hank grinned.

"How low class do you think I am?" I volleyed. "I save burping for at least date four."

We walked outside to the sidewalk. A barker was luring passersby into a bar to watch a fight on TV. I turned to Hank, my thighs backed against a low metal railing.

"So, what do you want to do, Hank?" I asked, holding his eyes.

Hank flicked his cigarette onto the street and closed the short distance between us.

"This," he said, his voice gravelly.

The kiss was surprisingly tender. His fingertips brushed my chin. I steadied myself against the railing. He tasted sweet, not like cigarettes at all. I felt the kiss burn slowly down me as if my lips were a wick he had sparked.

We agreed to take the train to his place, get his car, and drive to mine.

The nearest Metrorail station was a three-quarters of a mile walk. I think we held hands, but I don't remember. What I do remember is that every block or so, he would stop walking and kiss me. I also remember grinning and blushing every time.

The Metro platform was crowded, which seemed like a personal affront as we tried, sort of, not to claw at each other obscenely while we waited for the train to arrive. When the train doors opened, Hank slid onto a bench seat at the end of the car, facing a glass partition. The seat was snug for two people, so he pulled me onto his lap. I was facing him as we continued to make out.

I was covered in winter layers of a knee-length coat, sweater, pencil skirt, goldfish tights, and boots. This dissuaded Hank not a whit. Without me noticing how he managed it, he snaked his hand inside my coat, up my skirt, and between my legs, pressing against the damp V of my tights. I buried my face in his neck and breathed hard, as the train bumped along.

"This is me," he said and withdrew his hand. We bustled off the train and walked another half mile to his apartment, with the requisite kissing stops. I waited outside while Hank went inside for his car keys and to tell his wife his plans to drive me home. He returned with a short-haired, thirty-pound brown dog of indeterminate breed.

"I need to take her for a walk," he said.

I petted the mutt and tagged along. After the walk, Hank unlocked his Ford Bronco, and I climbed inside while he returned the dog to his apartment. My goldfish tights felt like bindings. I pulled off my boots and shoved my tights and panties inside one of them.

Hank got into the driver's seat and leaned over to kiss me. His thumb played with my nipple under my sweater, sending sparks down my spine. I shed my coat and climbed over the front and back seats to the very back.

"C'mon," I said.

Hank lumbered over, and his hand slid up my thigh under my skirt. I moaned. I could feel him hard under his jeans. I reached for his belt buckle, and he backed away.

"No, I don't want to do it here. Let's wait until we get to your place," he said.

I groaned and climbed back into the front seat, pulling my sweater and boots on as he started the car.

At a traffic signal, Hank stopped and grinned at me. "Well, look at that, a red light."

I raised an eyebrow. "Yes?"

"Come closer," he said, and I shimmied over. His kisses reached a tender spot inside me. They were unhurried, as if he knew exactly how long he had until the green light beckoned.

We reached my house several miles and kisses later. Will was asleep in his room. Eric and Marianne were in the guest room overhead. Hank followed me into the master bedroom, and I locked the door.

We tumbled onto the bed, throwing off our clothes. When the time came for protection, I saw two condoms and a small bottle of lube on the nightstand. I snickered. *Eric.* But Hank had brought his own. At the end of an afternoon and evening of drinking, Hank was not in the best shape to consummate the encounter, although we had a lot of fun trying.

After the fire was somewhat quenched, I wasn't sure if we even liked each other, or if it had been pure heat on both sides. When he said something about me coming out with him to a show the following weekend, I turned in bed to meet his eye.

"Say something nice," I dared him.

"When you first walked up to me on the street, I thought, *She's out of my league.*"

That was not what I had been expecting. Maybe it was a line, but it worked. He styled himself as a bad boy rebel in a pop-collar world. I was a white-collar professional in an occupation he disdained. This, I thought, could be interesting.

The next day, upon due consideration, some processing with Eric over eggs and coffee, and searching online for the show Hank had mentioned, I sent him a note. "Assuming you are not shaking your fist at the sky and demanding those twelve hours of your life back, yes, I would like to see that show you invited me to. It seems totally rad, and that's not just the slice of pizza as long as my arm talking."

The night of our second date, I was paralyzed with indecision about what to wear that would be hip enough but not look like I was trying too hard. Marianne was at the house before her date with Eric and she responded to my call for fashion help, reassuring me that I could rock black jeans, a tight shirt, and black boots. Hank and I entered the small theater from an alley and sat in the front row. We drank three-dollar cans of PBR as we witnessed a wacky cage fight meets burlesque meets Elvis impersonator, where the audience threw oversized fake amphetamines into a toilet on stage. In the last act of the show, the emcees announced an Elvis trivia contest. Before I knew it, Hank jumped on stage to compete, and damn if he didn't win. I laughed hard, spitting warm beer onto my boots. He bounced back into his seat, holding his prize coasters bearing the King's face and grinning wider than Charlie holding a golden ticket to Wonka's factory. I stopped laughing long enough for him to kiss me. What a night. I couldn't wait for more.

A few weeks later, Hank and I made plans to catch a burlesque show a friend of mine was in. We arrived early enough for the comedians' acts before the burlesque. Hank ordered a beer and a shot, and I said I'd have the same. The comedy was that cringe-inducing kind where you start to get embarrassed for the comics, so we bagged it, ordered another round of drinks, and went upstairs to explore.

The venue was an old movie house. On the top floor were the restrooms, a sofa, and an unmanned bar. We sat thigh to thigh on the sofa with our drinks in hand and our feet on an old coffee table. We were alone. Indecipherable rumblings from the stage drifted up.

Hank had accused me of not being forthcoming enough. Being new to polyamory, I was unsure how much to share, and it unsettled me. Hank appeared to be an open book, easily wearing a mantle of no shame in his game. I inhaled and, in a continuous sentence, I gave him the brief history of Natalie.

I had no stories to compete with his tales of childhood challenges, arrests, drug use, and copious sex, so I did not even try. We sipped our drinks and made out. After finishing our second round of drinks, we headed downstairs for the burlesque show. We ordered another round, and I gave a supportive shout to the emcee. Hank laughed and told me I was heckling; my inebriation seemed to amuse him.

The making out, the booze, and my lack of enthusiasm for seeing more of the titty show led me to propose we leave if we wanted to get to the more serious fooling around bit. It was midnight by then.

Going to Hank's place was rarely an option. We typically ended up at a hotel or my house. From the very start of our relationship, we were extremely sexual with each other, like a craving that needed sating. Sometimes, I felt that we did pre-sex stuff to convince ourselves that we could wait to paw each other, and so he could relate to his wife that we weren't only doing the horizontal mambo.

See, hon, we took in a movie / went to a show / played pool / had dinner / drove go-karts (and then screwed like rabbits). I sensed that Sylvia did not have a full picture of the amount of time we spent naked, but that information was his to share or not to share. Eric loved to hear as much as I wanted to tell him.

We drove to my house. I should say *he* drove because he always drove, often like a bat out of hell, always not wearing his seatbelt, and with one hand on his MP3 player or up my skirt, depending. I was not in the best condition to be behind the wheel and was hypervigilant about BAC levels and my bar license. Hank, on the other hand, was not affected by booze, being a vet at the drink and not slight of frame. He was six feet tall and at least 200 pounds.

I had the window down, enjoying the breeze, and was looking forward to wearing a lot less clothing in fifteen minutes.

He pulled into my driveway, and we quietly, *shh*, quietly ascended the steps.

Bedroom door closed, then locked. Boots, Chucks, his jeans, my skirt, and undergarments flung about in record time. Me on the bed. Him on the bed. Kissing, fondling, moaning, screwing. Bed spinning. What? Was the bed spinning? Ignore bed spinning. Screwing, yes, that's good. Oh, no. The ceiling shouldn't be sideways, should it? Final thrust. Climax. Uh-oh. Push him off. Run to bathroom. Grab the porcelain god and bow. Stomach contents, hello.

"You okay?" I heard from a few feet away.

Obviously not. More retching.

"You know, you shouldn't try to keep up with me. I've got a hundred pounds on you."

I heard the grin in his voice. Smug bastard.

I was beyond embarrassed. I was kind of crying, that's how stupid I felt. I mean, how fucking old was I, and I was puking up the bar tab like a rookie Tri-Delt? This early in our relationship, my springing from the bed and barfing into the toilet was not a visual I was thrilled to present.

"Would you hand me that robe, please?" I managed to whisper and point to the hook on the back of the door.

I wrapped myself in my fluffy, pale pink mom robe. Very sexy.

I avoided eye contact as I rinsed my mouth at the sink, and he hovered about, not certain how to help, but not all that ill at ease. I was sure he had seen a woman lose her cookies before. He had told me about a girl who threw up out the window of his car on their first date. I wasn't that bad. This was at least our fifth date.

I moved toward the bedroom. The room refused to stand still. The thought of doing anything but falling into bed and embracing unconsciousness seemed too onerous. I apologized like mad for the state I was in.

Hank chuckled at me. "I guess I'll see myself out?"

I was disappointed because hell if I didn't want a night of passion with him, but damn that ceiling refused to stay over my head in one spot. I hugged my terrycloth closer.

"Yes, please excuse me for not escorting you out," I said, "but fucking you makes me sick."

That drew a low laugh. He finished dressing and told me to drink lots of water and take aspirin. I don't know if I did. The room was still spinning the next morning when I awoke, although less so.

Eric had slept in the guest room with Marianne. He checked in on me in the morning, as was his way. I moaned against the sunlight and relayed the prior evening's events.

He laughed sympathetically. "I'm sorry the evening didn't turn out as you had hoped."

"I must have looked like a sophomoric idiot in front of Hank," I groaned.

Eric smiled, shook his head, and sighed at my vanity. "I'm sure that's not the case."

He brought me ginger ale and ibuprofen. He offered me breakfast.

"God, no!" I groaned.

He went to the kitchen to make some for himself, Marianne, and Will, if he was awake. Then, mercifully, he left me to sleep off the rest of the hangover.

In the afternoon, Hank texted to see how I was doing. He reminded me to avoid whiskey and to resist the competitive impulse to prove I was as hardcore as he was, because clearly I was not. I was just a girl who liked a guy and was doing what I thought I should to be a fun date.

I was also learning how to date as an adult while being true to myself. I was not a drinker. I was a two-and-a-half-glasses-of-anything gal. After that, the line between fun-time Natalie and passed-out Natalie was wafer thin.

Barring a booze overdose, fucking Hank never made me sick. It made me writhe and moan and even scream. I cried once or twice, and I'm sure I smiled a lot. But sick? Not a chance.

* * *

While dating Hank, I discovered I had a knack for sexy role-play. It started over texting and took on life in the bedroom. Once, I had called him "Mister" as a joke when he sounded like a teacher instructing a student, and it turned into a bit. He was good at developing a story via text. It was a silly, naughty diversion from work. I could visualize him as a young teacher wearing a white button-down, black tie, and Clark Kent glasses, and I thought it might be fun to carry out a teacher-student charade in person.

"I have the shirt and tie but no glasses," he said.

"I have a schoolgirl getup," I responded, "and I can find some glasses."

While Eric and I were at Party City on a Saturday afternoon, I looked for glasses for my date with Hank that night. I found a black plastic pair that was the right size and shape, but attached was a big flesh-colored nose.

I approached Eric with the plastic prop and sheepishly explained what I was looking for and why.

Eric threw his head back and laughed. "Let me see that." He examined the nose and glasses combo and said, "It should be easy to clip off the nose and make sure there are no sharp edges. I'll take care of it."

And he did. The glasses turned out to be the perfect on-the-nose accessory to Hank's shirt and tie. We had a great time with the role-play that night, and Eric was pleased that his handiwork had facilitated our fun.

* * *

By the time I was dating Hank, Eric and I had one living parent between us. My father's home was across the country, so I did not see a need to announce my relationship lifestyle. But my sister, who also lived far from me, was another matter. From the frosty morning my parents brought her home from the hospital, placed her gently in my three-year-old lap, and introduced me to my baby sister, Julia had been the best gift they ever gave me. I had preschool memories of pulling sticks out of her tiny fists that she was trying to put in her mouth, and later scowling at grown women in the library restroom when they told my short-haired, eight-year-old sister, "Little boys are not allowed in here."

"That's my sister," I spat, putting my arm around Julia.

I was reluctant to burden my little sister with my poly freakiness.

Julia often accompanied her husband to an annual out-of-town conference while his parents watched their kids.

"Do you go to the conference with him?" I asked her.

"No," she said. "I do my own thing and see him in the evening."

"What do you think about you and me exploring the city during the day and the three of us meeting for dinner at night?" I offered. "No kids, no responsibilities."

"Sounds great," Julia said.

"Meet you in St. Louis!" I said, and Sister Weekend was born.

During the first trip, Julia and I were waiting for my taxi to take me to my hotel when she said, "Can I ask you a question?"

"Yes," I said, "if you want an honest answer." Somehow, I knew.

"Do you have an open marriage?"

"Yes."

"Does Eric date?"

"Yes."

"Do you?"

"Yes."

"Is Eric seeing someone?"

"Yes, he's been seeing the same woman for more than a year." That was Marianne.

"Are you seeing someone?"

"Yes, for a few months." That was when I was besotted with Hank.

I was unsure how and when she had connected the dots. I suppose I left enough hints if anyone had cared to notice, and she did. I told her I was happy to answer her questions, but I didn't want to overwhelm her with information.

I tried to maintain my big sister, mom-like demeanor—our mother had been gone for twenty years by then—but inside, I was squealing: *Yay! Now, I can talk to Julia about my polyamory, share my dates, and reveal this new, glorious, scary, and fun part of my life with someone who means so much to me.*

Then I told myself, *Slow down, Natalie.* Julia—to my mild disappointment—was not as giddy at hearing my news as I was in sharing it. My sister needed processing time.

She asked, "Are you happy?"

"Yes!" I said, beaming.

She indulged me when I showed her photos of my new guy and teased me only a little when I told her how much younger Hank was.

Julia didn't probe me about my poly life during that trip or after. We had plenty to talk about—our kids' latest triumphs and challenges, bosses and colleagues who tested our patience, and when we would see each other again.

***

Attendant with dating Hank was my metamour relationship with his wife, Sylvia. We both had what hierarchical polyamorists called a *primary relationship* with our spouses. Hank's primary relationship was with Sylvia, and mine was with Eric. I was Hank's *secondary relationship*, and he was mine.

Polyamorists, swingers, and relationship anarchists have debated, and will continue to debate, the relative goodness, fairness, practicality, ethics, and effect of what many consider non-egalitarian relationship structures. I have seen a growing trend toward a rejection of hierarchical terminology such as "primary" and "secondary" over concern that some participants may be perceived as less important or valued. However, recognizing that a *nesting partner* (a partner you live with), or a spouse (a partner you are legally bound to), or a co-parent is inherently connected with you, in ways other partners are not, does not devalue other partners if you treat people with consideration. As the 2014 primer, *More Than Two: A Practical Guide to Ethical Polyamory* by Eve Rickert and Franklin Veaux, cautioned: Don't treat people as things.

I embraced my roles both as a primary and as a secondary partner. I found comfort in knowing my place in my relationships with Eric, Hank, and anyone else who came along. At long last, I saw with Hank the potential for what I thought I wanted—a secondary relationship with mutual affection and growth similar to what I envied in Eric's bond with Marianne.

I was determined to be The Best Secondary I Could Be! I resolved to be evolved, open, and embracing of my new metamour. I would respect Hank's familial and marital time and thus show respect to Sylvia. I would not usurp their primary relationship. Call him or incessantly text him during weekday evenings absent an emergency? No way. Distract him from his kid's music concert because I was feeling disregarded or ignored? Never. Accuse his wife of cockblocking me? Perish the thought.

Navigating the metamour arena was not intuitive. Let's face it, what bedtime story includes the Princess, her Prince, *and* the Prince's Wife/Girlfriend/Boyfriend/Lover/Other? I had no guide to tell me how this worked. In my childhood home, there was Mom, Dad, Me, Sister, Dog, and Hamster.

What was the model for metamour relationships?

I figured that friendship was a good starting point. Metamours are your partner's *other partners*—people you are civil with, possibly friendly toward, or even more. How that relationship evolves, or doesn't, is as variable as the people involved.

Marianne was my default metamour model. Because she and Eric spent so much time together at our house, Marianne's integration into our family happened quickly, and Will accepted her presence with minimal notice and apparent ease, despite not being told the full nature of his father's relationship with her.

For the family celebration of his fourteenth birthday, Will chose his favorite steakhouse and invited Marianne, who was at the house already. She wore her weekend uniform of jeans and a sweater, her honey hair in a ponytail. She wore no makeup, rocking a fresh-faced vibe.

The host sat us at a four-top. He then collected my son's wine glass and reached over to take the one at Marianne's place setting.

"Excuse me, I'm going to need that," she said as she looked up at him and placed her hand on his wrist. He released the glass.

I swallowed a laugh and caught Eric's eye. It was not a stretch to think Marianne and Will, both dark-eyed and brown-haired, were our kids. Later, the adults laughed about the Incident with the Wine Glass, debating whether our presumptive daughter resembled me or her father more.

In many ways, Marianne set the bar for polyamory excellence that I strived to emulate. The icy February following the birthday dinner, when Eric, Will, and I were driving home from Pennsylvania with my grandmother's piano in a U-Haul trailer, Marianne answered Eric's call to prep for our arrival. She shoveled our driveway, and when the bag of ice melt pellets ran out, she improvised by sprinkling all the table salt from the kitchen cabinets. Then she, our next-door neighbor, a friend, our son, and Eric hefted the old spinet inside. I supervised.

More and more, I appreciated Marianne's presence in our lives. I was eager to call upon my experiences with her to forge a positive relationship with Sylvia, who, unlike Marianne, was married like me, giving us a commonality that I thought would foster friendship. As I would come to realize, the complexities of the marriage of my new lover and his wife would remain a mystery to me.

Hank and Sylvia had been married two years when Hank and I started dating. It was his first marriage and her second. They had been together for a few years before that, some of that living several states apart because Hank moved to Washington to start a new job and get settled before Sylvia and her son followed. Sylvia had dumped Hank's best friend for him.

During the initial winter of our relationship, Hank and I were in a local motel room. It was our first chance to spend an uninterrupted evening getting to know each other's bodies. As we paused for breath after a session of intense, mutually satisfying fooling around, Hank had to satisfy another need.

"I'm going outside for a smoke," Hank said. He pulled on his black jeans, skipped his boxer briefs, slid into his Chucks, and shrugged on his leather jacket, his cigarettes and lighter in its pocket. The room door opened onto a second-floor exterior walkway.

When Hank came back inside, he shivered. "Damn, it's cold outside."

I looked up from the bed, where I was naked, but warm, under the covers. "Maybe you should quit smoking."

During the next post-sex smoke break, Hank saw a text from Sylvia. Hank's brow knitted and he mumbled, "Oh shit. I think I'm in trouble." After my reflexive irritation at the interruption, I raced to get dressed and practically pushed Hank out the door.

"You have to go home. Now," I said.

"But I didn't do anything," he half-whined.

"You must have done something," I said, "and I don't want to get on Sylvia's bad side before I even meet her. Let's go."

I didn't know, and Hank didn't volunteer, what was going on at his home that evening, but I figured the primary came first. If she texted him, it must have been important to her. For now, that was enough. I assumed that she respected his dating time as I respected Eric's, and she would not interrupt it without good reason.

The week after that motel date, Hank texted me "The Rules" to govern our relationship. I sensed that Sylvia was behind the enumerated decree, but I didn't ask.

(1) *No overnight dates without prior permission*. That seemed fair.

(2) *No out-of-town dates*. Hank noted that the rule could be amended or suspended, depending on the longevity of our relationship and whim of the primary (oops, sorry)—the agreement of all parties. This rule disappointed me because Eric had out-of-town dates on occasion, and I would have liked to have them, but it was too early in Hank's and my relationship for me to get twisted up about it.

(3) *No babies*. I could not stop laughing. Someone needed a specifically articulated rule that Hank and I would not have a child together? It took all my snark-suppression abilities not to send Sylvia a note that said, "Oh c'mon, Sylvia, just one baby? Hank and I would make a cute one. Pretty please?" When I shared that with Hank, to lighten the mood, he chortled.

But in all seriousness, I respected Sylvia and Hank for stating their (her?) rules early. Reading them let me know her concerns and how I could be The Best Secondary I Could Be! I understood the need for rules because I had made them for Lorraine.

I hooked my fifth digit into Hank's for a pinky swear, and that was that.

Two weeks later, Hank and I went out for a weekend lunch at a pizza and ping-pong joint about halfway between his place and mine. As we were finishing our pie, Hank got a call from his stepson.

"Okay," he said and ended the call. "The boy is going out with friends, and Sylvia is still with her boyfriend, so my apartment is empty."

"Oh yeah?" I kept my tone even.

"We could go to mine," Hank said. "I mean, if you want."

"Sure," I said. "I'd like to see your place."

Hank, Sylvia, and Owen—"the boy," as Hank always referred to him—lived in a two-bedroom, two-bathroom apartment.

"And this is the master bedroom," said Hank, gesturing through an open door.

I sat on the bed. "It seems nice and firm."

"You can't really know, though, can you?" Hank shrugged. "Until you test it."

"True," I said, playing my part.

So, we fooled around.

We were sitting on the living room sofa, fully clothed, with our feet on a black lacquered wooden coffee table that Hank had engraved with a red cobra insignia from a comic he liked, when Sylvia strode through the front door.

I immediately sat straighter, preparing to get up, introduce myself, and shake hands or hug or something.

Sylvia eyed us briefly and said to Hank, "I texted that I was on my way home."

"Sorry, I didn't see it," said Hank. "My phone is in my jacket."

Readying myself to leave, I reached for my leather jacket. Before I could speak or Hank could introduce me, Sylvia said abruptly, "I used to have a jacket like that."

I instinctively retracted my head a few inches as if a snake had hissed at me. No "Hi, I'm Sylvia. You must be Natalie. Nice to meet you." Then she turned away.

With her back to me, she spread out her beads and crafting purchases on a counter to display for Hank. I remained awkwardly on the sofa and waited until she was done talking to Hank about the baubles, so Hank could drive me home.

She offered no form of goodbye to either of us. My head bent, I walked out the apartment door, and Hank followed.

While Hank drove, Sylvia texted him about how much trouble he was in. I later found out that she was annoyed because she assumed he had kicked her son out of the house so he could "get laid"—her words—and that had not been preapproved. I could see how that would irritate her, if it were true, which it was not.

The impression she left with me, her new metamour, was that she was not a fan of me or Hank, at least in that moment. Hopefully, though, I thought, we could move past this little hiccup. Onward, ho.

* * *

Sylvia and I began sharing our experiences with polyamory via email, Sylvia's preferred method of communication.

"Poly was Hank's idea," Sylvia told me.

"I thought you had a boyfriend," I responded.

"I do," she replied. "I figured, why not. As long as Hank is going to date, I'm not going to be left out. You can be sure of that. We have been dating about two years. He is a generous lover."

Not that I asked, but good for you? Was that a dig at Hank . . . ?

I told Sylvia that I had been in an open marriage with Eric for years, starting with swinging, and had been dating on my own for about a year. "So far, my metamours have been Eric's girlfriends. I'm looking forward to us getting to know each other."

She wrote, "It sounds like you have more experience at this than I do. I am not sure why Hank wants to do this, except for more pussy, but I can go along with it for now, anyway. Maybe you can help me understand some of this poly stuff I get on the online chats and message boards sometimes."

"I'm not very familiar with the internet chat forums," I began, "but I've read some books on polyamory and listen to a practical podcast called *Polyamory Weekly*. I'm a huge fan of the host, Cunning Minx, and I can send you a link. My other metamour, Marianne, has been poly for years, and I sometimes discuss issues with her. I believe that communication is essential in polyamory, so I'm glad we're doing that."

I also talked to her about non-poly topics. "The gym is an invaluable mental escape from parenting and life chores and keeps me happier physically due to some back problems."

Sylvia wrote back, "I have been interested in trying a yoga class near me that meets on Wednesday nights. How about we take it together?"

Shit, I thought. My commute by train was usually reliable enough that if I left the office in time, I could be home to slip on my Lycra shorts and T-shirt, drive the four minutes to the gym, and attend a coveted core or Pilates class. Often, Eric would come with me and lift weights in a just-us routine I cherished. We could be home for a late dinner with Will.

Sylvia lived a thirty-minute drive from me, without traffic, and a weeknight commute would suck. Also, I did not like yoga.

I dreaded rejecting her idea for fear she would see it as a rejection of her, but I was so intent on being a good metamour that I considered committing to a bag of stress.

After a few drafts, I emailed her. "Hey, Sylvia, I wish that a midweek yoga class near you could work with my schedule, but I can't see swinging it. I would love to meet up for dinner on a weekend to relax and get to know each other. Pick a place you like."

Sylvia chose a casual restaurant downtown. The cramped table setup required us to sit on the same side of a bench seat. I had to keep turning my head to see Sylvia as we talked. It was awkward.

When the server left the bill on the table, I put my credit card on it.

"I'll get it," I said.

Sylvia was sitting on my left, and I was facing right. I thought I heard her say, "I'm not into you like that."

I turned to her. "What?"

"If you're expecting the two of us to get down because you're with Hank, that's not going to happen," she said.

"Whoa, Sylvia. I am not into women like that, and I am *not* coming on to you," I said. "I was just trying to be nice by paying."

Hank and I shared date costs. He might get dinner, and I would pay for the hotel room. My household made more money than theirs, so I paid for more. The thought of Hank spending his family's money on me made me uncomfortable.

Sylvia's shoulders relaxed. "Okay. Just so we are clear."

"Crystal." I laughed uncomfortably. *What the hell? Was no one ever nice to her unless they wanted something?* True, I wanted a good relationship with her, but the jump from platonic friendship to lesbian sex was a leap I did not see coming.

Even though we were not destined to be yoga buddies or lovers, all was not lost in my quest to be The Best Secondary I Could Be! In her initial messages to me, Sylvia looked to me for insight into polyamory, and I wanted to help. Perhaps I fancied myself as having something worthwhile to share. Perhaps I saw exchanging thoughts on polyamory as a pathway to connection. I even invited her to a local talk on metamours. That's poly-positive, right?

Sylvia and I sat on folding chairs in the back of a hotel conference room near Union Station. At the end of the talk, the speaker fielded questions about metamour relations. These questions included an old favorite, "How do I deal with feelings of jealousy and abandonment when my nesting partner is on a date?"

The speaker's response was one I had heard many times: "Value the time. Treat yourself to something you like to do, especially something your partner does not. It could be downtime streaming a show, a long bath, or seeing friends. Don't do chores. Think ahead to arrange reconnection time with your partner after their date."

The first time I heard the advice on a podcast, I thought it was a lot of whiny hooey, but I kept hearing the same suggestions from different people, so I tried some. I found value in post-date reconnection with Eric, even if it was simply a smile and kiss to tell me he was happy to see me. I nodded at the speaker and glanced at Sylvia.

Sylvia was rolling her eyes. At a restaurant after the talk, she said, "I can tell you that I am not pining for Hank while he's out. What a crock. If you signed up for poly, you should go out there and date."

"I get that, but it doesn't always work out that way," I said. "Haven't you ever been home alone when Hank was out and you didn't have a date and you felt out of sorts, or lonely, or envious? I know I have."

"I wouldn't let poly mess with me like that," she said.

I changed the subject.

* * *

Despite the challenges of my metamour relationship, I had a blast with Hank. We did wild things, at least wild for me. Sex in an alley, a movie theater, a federal park, or a car, anyone? We zipped up jumpsuits and sped around a racetrack. We devoured juicy Ray's Hell Burgers as big as our faces and Dangerously Delicious pies with buttery crusts. We attended plays, concerts, shows, clubs, and movies, and spent hours discussing books, debating politics, and sharing philosophies.

We had our little rituals, most of them initiated by Hank. We didn't text before our Saturday dates, heightening the anticipation. He kissed me at every stoplight, a charming ploy I suspect he'd been using since he could drive. We fooled around while he drove and while I drove. He made the same Scottish toast, whether we raised shot glasses or beer cans. "Here's to us! Who's like us? Damn few, and they're all dead." He knelt to pet every dog in our path. I beamed at his cooing, "Aren't you a good girl?"

* * *

The summer after Hank and I started dating, he and Sylvia took a much-anticipated ten-day vacation. Before the trip, Hank told me about their itinerary and the friends they would see.

"I'm happy that you guys will get to do some adventuring together. Have a great trip, Hank. I can't wait to hear about it when you get back."

"Thanks, Nat. I put a lot of work into planning. Can't wait to go."

At that juncture in our relationship, Hank and I messaged each other on and off throughout the day, and even sometimes after he got home at 3:00 p.m. I was in the throes of NRE, and if his constant engagement with me was any evidence, so was he. It was exciting and naughty. I was embarrassed to admit to Eric how much time I spent trading texts—and sexts—with Hank. I discovered that I was good at creating sexual scenarios in text. Hank would interject just the right number of responses to keep my narrative flowing. I locked my office door more than once while we finished the stories, and we each finished ourselves.

Hank texted me a few times during his vacation with Sylvia. One night, he was roaming the city alone because, he told me, Sylvia wanted to stay in the hotel room. He sent me a photo of graffiti he liked, and I responded briefly. I imagined he texted me because he was lonely and maybe even missed me or missed someone to share his nocturnal wanderings. After all, we were in the habit of chatting every day.

After their vacation, I received an email from Sylvia.*

> I don't think you will be seeing me soon.
>
> When Hank and I went on vacation, I was looking forward to getting away from everything associated with the here and now. It was our time, like how I don't contact him when he is on a date with you. You just couldn't respect that. As he pointed out, it's not how you and Eric do. You two go on vacations together and drag your tertiaries along in spirit. That's fine for you, but I've let you know that I stay out of the time you have with Hank out of respect, and you were aware of my expectations of him to be present with me when he is with me.

She also wrote:

> I also find out about completely private conversations between us that are shared with you. You don't share of yourself with me, and I let you have that privacy and do not nose around for it—but I don't get afforded the same from either of you. Instead, y'all get together and discuss what Sylvia is going through right now as though I can't and shouldn't be able to work out my own personal feelings with myself or in the safety of the intimacy I thought I shared only with my husband.

* The email exchanges with Sylvia are substantially verbatim with minor edits for grammar, punctuation, clarity, and brevity.

> It doesn't occur to either of you to bring ME into these conversations, which is odd because when he did the same about long past personal situations of yours, I felt it invaded you in a way I could [not] allow to be unknown to you. I told you what I knew. You do not afford me the same courtesy. Nope.
>
> At this point, y'all can continue seeing each other, but he isn't to share anything about me to you, and I no longer want to know you. Your correspondence with him will be on his time and not our time. And in the future, if he is out of town with me, have more respect for that and recognize that he isn't available to you at those times.

After reading Sylvia's 9:56 a.m. email, I was shaking at my office desk when I responded at 10:13 a.m.: "Wow. I don't know what is going on, but I do know that hurt, and I did not deserve that. When I calm down, I'll try to figure it out."

I was upset because my metamour hated me. I was upset because I was an awful metamour. I was upset that she had attacked me over assumptions that were, in fact, wrong.

And I was upset with Hank, our shared partner. Hank neither gave me a heads-up that Sylvia was pissed, nor came clean to her about how he had initiated communication with me. I was learning that Hank felt his balls retract when the women in his life were unhappy, so he took the path of perceived least resistance—or self-protection. I suspect Sylvia had told him she wanted this vacation just for them with no girlfriend contact. If I had been made aware, I could have been on board with a no-contact rule if she needed it or negotiated a weekly check-in. I doubt she knew that Hank and I talked every day for hours. Cold turkey was a big ask.

Before I could text Hank with *WTF is going on?*, finish my workday, feed my family, tell Eric why I was on edge, and gather my thoughts, Sylvia responded:

> Oh, you don't need to try to figure it out. I AFFORD YOU that respect. You sat on information about the HERE and NOW concerning my own husband. Is it information I would have shared with someone as they and

> I built a rapport of sharing private moments and vulnerabilities like two peers would do? YUP. But you don't share yourself with me in that way.
>
> I was going to have a talk with you about your lack of opening up to me—whose husband you're fucking—about things you deal with in your own life despite me not fucking your husband. He did tell me once that he took a problem we were having to you, and I reminded him that he insists I would just be wasting my time if I took our problems to anyone but him. I also told him that you don't open up to me, it was starting to make conversation with you a real drag, and I was losing interest in a friendship with you. You can't even open up to someone who isn't fucking your husband, but I'm supposed to be an open book to you?

I tried to recall what Hank had shared with me that would have upset Sylvia so much that I deserved nothing more than disposal.

I knew from Hank that his marriage often left him sleepless. When we started our daily chats with "Hey, how is your day going?" and Hank would say, "Eh, I didn't sleep last night because Sylvia and I were up all night, fighting," I would lend an ear to whatever he wanted to share. Many times, he would brush me off and we would talk about other things, but as his girlfriend, I hated to see him suffer. I would offer "Aw, baby" or "I'm sure you guys will work it out" or "Damn, that sounds rough." Sometimes he would vent with more specifics, and I would listen, but he rarely accepted advice when I tried to help around the edges, careful not to overstep, with my suggestions to communicate better or listen more.

I was giving myself an ulcer debating how to respond to Sylvia. On the one hand, I wanted to expose my belly like a submissive animal to show she was alpha and that I would take her berating as long as she did not veto my relationship with her husband. On the other hand, I wanted to tell her to fuck off and that I hoped the boulder-sized chip on her shoulder crushed her as it crushed me.

While indecision wracked me, Hank messaged. "Sylvia told me, 'Oh, she has time to screw my husband, but not time enough to respond to me?'"

Eric thought I should ignore her obvious anger and refuse to engage in emotional ping-pong. "Write a short response."

"I don't know what to do," I said. "I want to appease her and not lose Hank. I want to acknowledge her concerns, but I don't want to be a simp."

Eric placed his hands on my shoulders. "Natalie, she sounds irrational. You don't have to respond to everything she wrote in that tirade."

I stayed up late crafting a response. I ended my email by telling her: "I did not intentionally disobey the rules or cause you pain. And, if I did, I AM SO VERY SORRY. If you have more to dish out at me, I will try to take it. But I really do hope our next round [ding!] will be less bloody."

Sylvia listened to my response and believed me about Hank texting first. She concluded Hank was not completely forthcoming, as in, *"Ah, Hank did not tell me that."* She even apologized for blaming me when she did not have all the facts.

I threw my hands up and danced. I was not the worst metamour ever! I could make this work.

Miscommunication—in Hank's case, non-communication—triggered unnecessary poly drama. When I confronted Hank about throwing me under the bus driven by his wife, with whom I was trying to find connection, he moaned, "I am just trying to keep everyone happy."

"Well, you didn't make either of us happy. Please stop trying to manage our emotions by keeping things from us that affect our relationship with each other and with you. How can we be legit friends if your actions put us in opposite corners of a boxing ring?"

"I have weed brain," he said, not for the first time, referring to his daily habit since he was an adolescent. "I don't remember stuff."

I rolled my eyes. Inexperienced with drugs, I didn't know how much to buy his defense. "There are only so many times that excuse will fly."

The following week, I received a package from Sylvia containing two boxes. One was a tube pan for baking cakes with a heart-shaped center, and the other pan made cakes with a checkerboard pattern. I was touched and immediately sent her a note of thanks. She remarked that if some people had wish lists, they wouldn't keep receiving cake pans. Hank's Amazon wish list had over two hundred assorted items, ranging from ten-dollar books to three-hundred-dollar gaming systems. The only mystery to him was which item Sylvia or I would choose.

Sylvia knew that creating cakes for people had been a hobby of mine ever since Will started having birthday parties. A month after the vacation dust-up and her apology gifts, I hosted a birthday party for Hank and suggested to Sylvia that she and I make the cake. I wanted to do something nice for Hank and include Sylvia in a celebratory kitchen table polycule event.

Hank had a phobia of octopi, so we made a squid cake with solid black eyes that we knew would freak him out. I thought a joint project and time together before the guests arrived would help us connect.

Sylvia brought ingredients for her pizza recipe. Eric hung a donkey piñata I picked out at Party City from a backyard tree. Hank's laughing face as Eric swung the ass just out of bat's reach made me smile, remembering that Eric had served in the same role at Will's ninth birthday party. So often Hank was an oversized kid, full of pure joy in the moment. I loved that about him.

Eric made a habit of including our partners and their partners in our lives, so I invited Sylvia and Hank to events that Eric and I planned to attend. I became reticent in extending those offers after Sylvia's emails made me start like a skittish rabbit, but I was still trying to be The Best Secondary I Could Be!

Ten months into my relationship with Hank, I invited them both to a Halloween party at a dance club Eric and I frequented. Sylvia, an accomplished seamstress, proudly assembled a sexy vampire costume with beaded earrings evocative of blood drops. Hank wore a shirt soaked in fake blood. He looked like he had been stabbed in the gut. Despite the gruesomeness of his costume, Hank's mischievousness was seductive. His perpetual state of slight dishevelment—in stark contrast to Eric's crisp lines and thoughtful attire—drew me to him.

After an hour at the club, drunk Hank kissed me. While I would have loved to feel his lips on mine longer, it would have pushed Sylvia's "I am your date, not hers" button. I reminded him of that and pushed him away, but she saw the kiss. She expressed her irritation to Hank at home later. Predictably, I got an email from her telling me how they had fought about it, and she had withheld sex as punishment.

At Eric's urging, I invited Hank and Sylvia to a spring showing of dozens of local artists called Artomatic. Then Eric got sick. I joked to Hank via text that Eric had a "man cold," a reference to a British video that kept Eric and me in stitches at its depiction of men acting like babies when they are sick, and women keeping on keeping on.

"It's a cold, not cancer," said Eric. "Go without me. I have tissues and NyQuil. I'll be fine."

So, I did. I was looking forward to seeing my boyfriend and my metamour and introducing them to my friends. Hank and Sylvia didn't show up. The next day, Hank told me they ghosted me for "reasons" he did not want to explain.

Much later, Sylvia told me, in one of her long emails, that she had imposed on a colleague to trade shifts only to find out that I was going solo. She had interpreted "man cold" as code for "faking sickness." She was livid and refused to attend. She thought I concocted the man cold ruse to see Hank and to screw her—not literally—by making her anticipated double date a threesome. Sylvia's machinations dizzied me.

On another occasion, Eric, Will, and I were invited to a crab feast at Hank and Sylvia's home. I was pleased to be included and looked forward to meeting their friends. I took it as a positive sign that Will was invited. Hank had advised me early in our relationship that Sylvia did not want his other partners' kids to become friends with Owen for fear that her fourteen-year-old would suffer unspecified trauma after Hank and his partner broke up and ended any friendships her son had formed.

At their party, Hank and Sylvia didn't introduce my family to their friends. I didn't know if I should introduce myself as a friend or a partner, which made me feel awkward and anonymous. I didn't want to out my hosts as polyamorous to any guests who didn't know. I didn't want to violate secret boundaries and incur Sylvia's ire. I would have taken the lead of my hosts, but whenever I looked for them, they were engaged with other guests, smoking, or laughing.

After we three had eaten and tried to chat with some strangers, I caught Eric's eye as he twirled his index finger in the air and tapped his watch, the signal for "Let's wrap this up and go." I collected Will, and we said our goodbyes. In the driver's seat, Eric was stone-faced and silent.

"It was nice of them to invite us over," I said with forced cheerfulness. "The crab legs were good, and the potatoes were just right. So tender."

Eric's eyes were fixed on the road. Will was in the back seat playing a handheld video game with his headset on.

"I know you don't like to eat crab legs because of the mess," I said, "so thanks for coming with me."

"Natalie, I am happy to support your relationship with Hank, but I don't like to see your partner and his wife being rude to you and our family. Have they never had partners over before—or had anyone over?"

Their lack of social graces irritated Eric, who unfailingly greeted our houseguests with warmth and introduced our friends to each other, pointing out something they might have in common to start their conversation.

"I don't know what to say, Eric. I don't think it was intentional. Not everyone is as comfortable playing host as you."

"Natalie, Attila the Hun would be a better host than those two, especially Sylvia. I couldn't wait to leave."

"Yeah, I got that from you, loud and clear," I said.

"I have trouble parsing any kind of positive vibe from Sylvia toward you," Eric said. "I know how hard you're trying."

"She's trying, too," I said. "I just have to be patient and remember that poly was hard for me, too."

Sylvia and I continued to work on our friendship. Whenever Sylvia had her hair cut blocks from my office, we would meet for lunch. We also chatted online, but our interactions felt awkward and forced when they involved Hank. Conversely, when we talked about poly in general, girl stuff, or parenting, our connection was less strained. That we both had romantic relationships with the same guy acted more as a barrier than as a bridge to our friendship.

A year after Hank and I began dating, Sylvia sent me a lengthy email, which, per usual, I read multiple times to decipher. The crux of what she wrote is in this excerpt:

> Hank downplays everything on his side of this. Some of his reasons are valid, but most of them are based on his bad past habits formed in his own dysfunctional childhood; fear of honesty and the punishment it always earned him. I can tell when he isn't being completely honest. I had nothing

> else to do but remember how guilty I felt with my boyfriend Jared and feel there must be something going on with you that Hank felt I'd be crushed by. You had an "alright time"? It was "okay"? Seems to be going on a while for you to just find it "alright" and "okay." It started to crack my head open.
>
> My dates with Jared involved getting a hotel room for the privacy it afforded us. I held nothing back from Hank, even if it might make him cringe at my description of our dates. I asked if he felt that we had been behaving in a way that indicated I was not honoring my primary connection with him. He was quiet for a while.
>
> Finally, he admitted that it was pretty damn close to how his night with you had gone. It was a huge relief that he didn't expect I'd have because all the guilt over my relationship with Jared disappeared.

As part of another email more than a year after Hank and I started dating, Sylvia wrote: "I don't want to be around Hank much the day after date night with you. I know the definition of compersion; I just don't feel it. It's better when the next day after your date night is a day I work because I can spend the next 8 hours away from him."

When Hank told me he slept on the sofa after he drove home from our dates, I thought he was avoiding waking Sylvia, who worked early on Sundays, but no. She couldn't stand the sight of him after he was with me. He cowered on his couch rather than sleep in the room I paid for. We skulked off at 2:00 a.m. like vampires shunning daylight.

For a year, Sylvia had no idea how much we were naked together. We shook the bedframes at the motel where I racked up loyalty points with each Saturday night visit. Our physical chemistry was a fundamental part of our relationship. I reveled in the fun we had before we dragged ourselves out of bed on predawn Sunday.

For a year, I wondered why the Rules banned hotel sleepovers. I yearned to wake up with my lover and have breakfast together. Eric had that. If the sight of Hank on Sundays irritated Sylvia, why not stay with me? Hank would say, "Reasons."

What Hank did not tell me, but Sylvia shared, was that when she was dating Jared, who lived alone, Hank did not want her sleeping at his house. When Hank started dating me, she insisted that what was good for the goose was good for the gander, never mind the impact on me.

"Fair is fair," Sylvia said. "Nothing personal, Natalie."

But it was personal. I was not party to their decision even though it affected me. I wasn't even dating Hank when the no-sleepover rule was made. It didn't seem fair. It seemed mean. Hank and I were in hierarchical polyamory structures because, as married couples whose lives were intertwined with our spouses in multiple ways, that made sense. Nonetheless, Eric and I strove to respect our secondary partners' agency and treat them with consideration, not as disposables.

As I struggled to be The Best Secondary I Could Be!, I felt that Sylvia and I spoke different languages and that she and Hank excluded me from decisions that affected me. While I tried to stay positive, I cringed at being a sacrificial pawn in their game of relationship chess.

Too often, being Sylvia's metamour sent my texting fingers flying to the group chat with my indispensable trio of friends who listened to my insecurities, venting, and moon-faced coos with equal parts comfort, reality-check, and "you go, girl!" encouragement. Rae was married and poly. Trisha was single and monogamous. Fiona was married and monogamous. All loved to dance, which was how our lives initially converged—at the local goth night that Eric promoted when Will was a baby.

"That sucks," said Fiona, when I told the girls of the latest challenge.

"Is he worth it?" asked Trisha. "There are better guys out there."

"Poly is tough, hon," said Rae, always the diplomat. "It sounds like you are doing your best with a difficult situation." She had weathered her own metamour storms, often with more grace than me.

"Thanks for listening," I responded. "I feel better getting it off my chest."

"We've got you," chimed in Trisha. "Whatever you decide. We love you."

On one rare occasion, Hank and I planned an overnight date with prior approval from Sylvia. We were to attend a Halloween event, complete with costumes in our suitcases and a pricey prepaid hotel room above the venue. At the hotel, not yet in our costumes, Hank received an email from Sylvia. He read it to himself on his phone, and his face dropped.

"Something wrong?" I asked.

He told me that Sylvia had announced that they could remain married, but they would each do as they pleased, and she would not wear her wedding ring anymore.

I was startled. "What are you talking about? What happened?"

"Before I left home to pick you up, we were fighting," Hank said. "She wanted me to stay home. I told her that would not be fair to you, so I refused."

I was fuming inside at what I saw as her gall to intrude on my date. I was surprised that Hank had refused to cancel our date because I was not used to feeling that our time together was more important than Sylvia's wants.

"I don't know what to do. This email is awful. I'm afraid for my marriage." He ran his fingers through his hair.

Hank was more distraught than I had ever seen him. He looked as if he might cry as he bent his neck over his phone, reading more of what appeared to be a long email. I was familiar with those.

"If you think you need to go home to save your marriage, then of course, do so," I said evenly.

I was irritated, but I downplayed it to Hank. Our date was ruined. Halloween was ruined. Eric was out with his girlfriend. I would be going home to an empty house to fume.

"I am sorry, really, but I have a terrible feeling that if I don't go home, I may not have a marriage."

"Can you drive me home first?" I asked. "It's Halloween. I don't know if I'll be able to get a cab." I lived five miles from the hotel.

We packed up our things and put our half-eaten delivery dinner in the trash. He pulled his car around from the garage while I checked out at the front desk.

On the ride home, he offered to pay for the hotel room.

"No," I said, "I don't want to take food out of your family's mouths. I can cover it."

"It's my money, dammit. I can pay for the hotel," Hank snapped. "I work a job I hate so Sylvia can play with plants. She doesn't make enough to cover my bar tab." Sylvia worked at a nursery, a job she enjoyed. She had given me a creative arrangement with a stunning magenta orchid as its centerpiece several months earlier. Hank figured at least one of them should like their job.

That was the first time I had heard Hank speak disparagingly about supporting Sylvia. We were silent for most of the ten-minute drive to my house.

I retrieved my suitcase and said, "I hope you work it out with Sylvia. I'm here if you need me."

"Thanks," he said. "Again, I'm sorry."

Sylvia's response to my email request to have my time with Hank respected cryptically referenced childhood issues she was dealing with at age thirty-nine. She told me that "your intimacies with Hank are not as important to me as my relationship with him and my need for him to be with me through this."

Aye aye, Cap'n, saluted The Best Secondary I Could Be!

* * *

About a year after Hank and I had started dating, Sylvia was seeing Leo. She had broken up with Jared a few months after I met her. Sylvia only dated single guys.

"I don't understand why anyone would date a married guy. You could never be queen bee," Sylvia told me during one of our chats.

I felt slapped, but I was still trying to be The Best Secondary I Could Be! so I just said that I respected the primary-secondary dynamic, and as long as all the players also respected it, the secondary would not be treated poorly.

Sylvia and Leo had been dating for a few months. He was unmarried and dated only Sylvia. At one of our lunches over ramen, Sylvia announced, "Leo said 'I love you.' I haven't told Hank yet. I am not sure how he will take it."

"I see." I choked a little on my noodles. Hank and I had been dating a year, and nothing close to those three words had been exchanged between us.

"How do you feel about it?" I asked.

"I don't know." She shrugged. "It seems a bit much, you know? We haven't been dating that long."

She disregarded his declaration as a juvenile infatuation because Leo was fifteen years younger than her. I disagreed. Sylvia was still thinking about how to respond to him.

Several weeks after our lunch, Sylvia confided that she was thinking of telling Leo that she loved him too. Given her past comments, I was a little surprised. I was also happy—for them as a couple, and for Sylvia that she had come to embrace polyamory by being open to sharing her heart with someone. I thought it was a big step to tell someone other than your spouse that you loved them when you had identified as monogamous for so long.

Sylvia was concerned about Hank's reaction. I hoped Hank would be the mature polyamorist I saw him as. I remember feeling a jolt the first time I heard Eric and Marianne express their love for each other, but I realized I didn't feel threatened. It was more that I wasn't prepared for the exchange, even though it was the natural progression of their relationship. I came to see it as tender—and enviable.

Before she met with Leo, Sylvia told Hank that she was going to tell Leo how she felt. I was heartened that Sylvia prudently deduced that Hank might need some reassurance and extra care . What I—and maybe she as well—did not predict was the intensity of his reaction.

"Hank slammed dishes around the kitchen," Sylvia reported. "He said he was 'fine' with whatever I wanted to do, but that, going forward, it would dilute the meaning of the words 'I love you' when I said them to him. That didn't sound to me like he was 'fine.'"

I blinked.

When had Hank come to hold this view, or had he always felt that love was a zero-sum game? Perhaps his reaction stemmed from his discomfort with expressing love. According to Sylvia, it was hard for Hank to say the words due to damage done in his childhood by his parents using love as a bartering stick. It had taken him two years to say it to her, the woman he would marry.

I found myself wondering if Hank viewed polyamory merely as his way to screw around with approval, or at least with tacit deniability.

A week later, I was having afternoon coffee with Hank when Sylvia and Leo's exchange of these words of affection came up.

"He's so young, and he's never been in a relationship other than with someone else's wife. How could he possibly know what love is?" Hank scoffed.

When I looked across the table, I saw a jealous, insecure, and not very polyamorous boyfriend. The jealousy and insecurity I understood, but his expression of how his wife's love for another minimized her love for him pained me. Furthermore, he made her feel bad for having those feelings and expressing them.

Why did this throw me so much? I thought I knew.

Several weeks earlier, Hank, a comic book freak from youth, had offered to take Will to the Free Comic Book Day that occurred each May. He, his stepson Owen, and Will would make a dude outing of it. I was touched that he had invited my son. Will was psyched. Owen, quiet and sullen the few times I met him, knew his mom and stepdad had an open marriage, but he never told Will. Our kids interacted only a few times.

Pickup time was wicked early on a Saturday, and I groused to Eric about having to be presentable when Hank arrived. Eric rolled his eyes and said, "Natalie, he isn't going to care what you look like. He loves you. Wear your bathrobe if you want." So I did.

The weeks following that May morning got me thinking about the 800-pound gorilla in the room: Love. My first thought was *Ha! No, no way. That's not how we are. You, my dear husband, may roll that way with Marianne, and more power to you both, but Hank and I are not the same.*

Did I drop the subject? Did I trust my instincts about the nature of my relationship with Hank?

Did Jesus eat pork rinds?

What I did was write to help myself think.

Eric and I said "I love you" to each other effortlessly, but I had never said the words to another guy. As I wrote, I thought about what love meant to me.

It started with a deep affection. It grew into concern for someone else's happiness and well-being so much that you were willing, and did at times, put their happiness before your own. For me, being with my beloved made me want to be a better person and brought out a better me. Loving someone meant feeling their pain and yearning to ease it. It was wanting to do all you could to make the other person happy and fulfilled.

If that was love, then yes, I loved Hank. Alone in my room, I tested the words out loud. They didn't burn my tongue.

That summer, I proposed to Hank that we go away for a long weekend. Eric had taken girlfriends on trips—to a West Virginia cabin and a Delaware beach with Marianne for a weekend; to Germany with Lorraine for a week. I had never been in a relationship where out-of-town excursions were on the table. I had a bounty of chits I could cash in with Eric, and after a year and a half with Hank, I thought I had demonstrated my goodwill and trustworthiness to Sylvia. Perhaps she would grant us dispensation. Rule Number Two specified no overnights without approval, to be applied for in advance, with a memorandum of reasons therefore, and to be granted rarely if ever.

Sylvia did not reject the proposal out of hand, so Hank and I discussed trip options. Going away was already a little uncomfortable because I had offered to finance the trip to impact his family economics as minimally as possible and be spared wifely wrath.

Discussing where to travel brought no concrete suggestions from him. In fact, the proposal was beginning to feel like an obligation that I was regretting I had suggested. If Hank had said, "Look, let's just skip it because I feel uncomfortable with you paying," I would have almost been relieved, even though I had been looking forward to my first getaway with my first poly boyfriend.

I had offered an adventure, and he viewed it as a burden—at least, that's how it came across to me. I felt a little like *I'm paying for this trip; the least you can do is suggest some options, so I don't have to do all the legwork. It's not as if I don't have a job and a life you know, while you spend hours surfing the net at work. Why not surf for vacation ideas?*

After dinner, driving to the hotel to fool around before going out to a movie—did I mention our dates included a lot of fooling around?—tears rolled down my cheeks.

Naturally, Hank asked me what was wrong. I shook my head and said nothing. I was trying to figure it out myself. Why exactly was I crying? What I came up with was: "You don't care enough about me or our relationship. I don't want to talk about this because I don't see the point. If I'm right, then we'll break up, and I don't want that. If I am being silly and paranoid, I'll feel stupid and vulnerable." I said none of that.

After he stopped the car in the hotel parking lot, he said, "Natalie, tell me. I can see you're upset."

I smiled. "I'm fine, really. I don't know why I am being this way."

He was not fooled because only a moron would have been. He was not a moron, but he stopped asking.

At the hotel, we started our typical groping. No matter what, we always seemed to be hot for each other. But it nagged at me, and while we were horizontal, I really started crying with not just tears, but with gasps and a dripping nose.

After the sex, I said, teary-eyed, "You're a bastard, Hank, but I love you."

Hank said, "Aw, that's sweet of you to say."

I felt emotionally drained as we fell asleep in each other's arms. I woke up and looked at the clock. It was 2:00 a.m. I was tempted to let Hank sleep, but I knew Sylvia would be annoyed if he wasn't on their couch when she awoke.

I touched Hank's arm and said, "We should probably get going."

A few days later, our texting chat had him saying everything *but* "I love you."

"I care about you. Isn't that the same thing?" he said.

"Then why not just say it?" I asked.

"Maybe I only have room in my heart for Sylvia," he said.

Sure, I was a little hurt, maybe more irritated than hurt, because who doesn't want to hear that the person they love loves them back? I wasn't made of stone. I resolved not to take his lack of mirroring as an insult, but . . . we had seen each other at least once a week for eighteen months. My expression of love could not have been a surprise to him.

I mentally kicked myself for falling prey to Eric's interpretation of my relationship with Hank. I was disgusted with myself for wanting what Eric seemed to have so easily that I ignored the truth of what Hank and I shared, or at least, what Hank shared with me.

I didn't tell Hank what a hurdle it had been for me to say "I love you" to him.

That's why, hearing Sylvia relate Hank's un-poly view of Leo's ardor over our lunch, after I had just expressed my love to him, felt like a sucker punch. How could Hank fail to see how his judgment of Leo would sound to the ears of his girlfriend, who had just braved the same declaration? I had clamped my mouth shut and drunk my tasteless coffee.

Later that day, I beat the horse again, poor nag, and sent Hank a message letting him know that his reaction to Leo led me to conclude he must think I was a lovesick puppy. I wanted him to understand that I had realized yes, it was true, we could have romantic love for more than one person at a time and that I, for one, was on board with the *amory* in polyamory. One love took nothing away from other loves, and I would not be made to feel wrong or deviant for expressing it to my boyfriend or anyone else.

I could not help but feel that something had changed; that Hank felt an imbalance in the Force or an obligation. I felt it, too. We argued over something petty and forgettable a month later. We made up, but I foresaw the end and started to disengage. I pushed him, almost daring him to break up with me. I couldn't bring myself to do it. He was my first in so many ways.

I had started seeing someone else earlier that summer, three months before Hank and I were to take our weekend getaway to New York. Lee was a married poly guy who had messaged me on OkCupid.

When I told Hank about Lee, he joked about his "replacement."

"Don't say that," I said.

At the time, I had meant it. No one was replacing anyone. I doubted that Hank understood that, to me at least, polyamory meant more than one love. If I had been on my game, I would have said to him, "Now that you mention it, Hank, would you show Lee how you do that thing with your tongue that I like so much? That would be over the moon."

Lee had invited me to a poly-friendly cookout, and Eric had encouraged me to invite Hank to foster polycule connectivity. I tried to be nonchalant in broaching the subject with Hank.

"Lee and his wife are having a poly cookout," I said. "They call it a poly-cue. Want to come with me?"

"Let me see what's on the calendar," Hank said.

"Sylvia is invited too, of course," I added quickly. "Marianne is coming."

"I'll let you know."

He didn't let me know.

In August, Hank and I drove to New York City for the weekend. We walked miles exploring the city, Hank reminding me to look up to take it all in, and that's how I found a second-story comic book store. We dined at an underground Japanese restaurant blocks from the Lower Manhattan courthouse depicted on *Law and Order* and saw Andrew Wyeth's *Christina's World* at the MoMA. We ate Hungarian hamburgers and, of course, pizza by the slice.

We had sex once in three days and went to bed early most nights. Naked beside him, I struggled to sleep. Was he losing interest in me?

"What's up? I was looking forward to using the toys in my bag," I said.

"We can have sex any time," he said. "I'm tired."

On our last night in New York, we had a silent argument, meaning I was silent, and he racked his brain for what he had done wrong. Whatever I wanted from him, from our relationship, I wasn't getting it. My sister Julia called while I was in line for food at a travel plaza on the drive home on Sunday. Feeling fatalistic, I told her that Hank and I were likely headed to done.

After we got home, we had another stupid argument that I engineered for no good reason except to test his affection. Not surprisingly, he failed. I think I knew that would happen. With the turmoil in his primary relationship, why would he want a pouty, unpredictable girlfriend? The differences between us, which I used to find stimulating, became tedious. I started resenting his political and philosophical views to an irrational extent.

A week or two later, he messaged me. "I'd like to have a meeting."

I thought, *There's a first. Are we a corporate board?*

I saw Hank's text while driving to see Lee. When I didn't immediately respond to Hank's request, he sent another text about how it was hard enough to prepare for a "serious talk" without me ignoring him. In an era of instantaneous communication, failure to do so was a hanging offense, so I texted Hank from Lee's driveway.

Three days later, Hank drove to my house. Eric had taken Will with him to give us space. I fostered hope that Hank and I would have a candid talk about our relationship. I imagined hot makeup sex after a cathartic discussion at my purposefully empty house.

When Hank arrived, he remarked about preferring more "neutral territory." What did he think was going to happen, a Mafia hit? But, considering Sylvia's violent tendencies during their arguments, including smashing their furniture, yelling so much that the neighbors called the cops, I could see the basis for what seemed to me to be laughable paranoia. Her dispute resolution methods, paired with her habit of driving at breakneck speeds through wealthy residential neighborhoods, daring anyone to challenge her, were disturbing.

I invited Hank to sit down on the back porch. He sat and lit a cigarette. Looking serious across the table, he slid a Jackson over.

"For the smokes you bought me," he said. Then he rambled on with vagaries about how we weren't communicating, and he had thought a lot about it, and he couldn't change stuff about me he wasn't cool with. "But I like you as a person, and I want to be friends."

I made a stab at drawing out more specifics to see if we could have a two-way discussion, intercourse without the in-and-out bit. In my head, I was thinking about how Eric and Marianne had been on the verge of breaking up more than once, but they talked and worked through it.

What I got from Hank was, "I don't want to sit here and make nasty judgments about you."

"Nasty judgments?" I asked. "You tell me you want to be friends, but you are holding nasty judgments about me?" I could feel my body temperature rise, and I wondered if my face was red.

I was thinking, *Fuck you, fuck you, fuck you.*

I said, "I have a lot of friends, Hank. I don't need more. You can't wave your hand and subtract sex from our relationship equation and still have a relationship. It doesn't work like that."

"That hurts that you don't want to be friends," he said.

"It hurts me that you hold nasty judgments but refuse to share them, while professing to like me 'as a person,' whatever that platitude means," I shot back.

Did he mean he liked me as a person as opposed to an aardvark or robot, or maybe an alien, or—oh, I know, a zombie!

"You can go now," I said.

He walked away, shoulders slack.

I sent him a note a day or so later telling him I wished him well, I bore him no ill will, and I treasured our time together. He said he meant it about being friends. I said no thanks to the consolation prize of membership in the Former Lovers But Now Just Friends of Hank Club.

Then the real fight began on a messaging site, because you should always engage in confrontational arguments virtually, where you cannot see facial reactions or gauge emotions.

Me: What is so wrong with enjoying each other physically but disagreeing about whether communism can work or Walmart is the Devil? It's exhausting.

Him: If you were going to treat me like a whore, you should have bought me nicer things.

Me: Are you serious?

Him: I could use some more video games and new clothes for instance.

Me: Are you for real saying you think I used you for sex?

Him: It sure sounds that way, doesn't it?

Me: I cannot believe you. I tell you all the time how intelligent you are, how I respect your opinion and perspective, and how I have grown from our discussions. Don't we spend hours a day talking about politics, books, and society? What about all the shows we went to, coffee chats, burgers and pie, and exploring the city on our bikes?

I spared him the reminder of all the hours I spent listening to him process the latest transgressions of his father, wife, stepson, employer, exes, or best friend. I did not mention all the times he typed his messages in capital letters to express his anger at someone or something because I did not regret those hours. It was part of being in a relationship. I was glad to offer him comfort or support. It was as if he had double-deleted the file that held our nonsexual engagement and my emotional support.

Him: You say that, but I feel like you did all that so you could get to the sex. Like eating your vegetables just to get dessert. You don't seem engaged when I try to talk about big things that matter to me, but rather, it's like let's hurry this up, so we can rip each other's clothes off already. That's what makes me feel like a whore.

Me: Please stop using that word. It's offensive.

Him: I think it's an apt description.

Me: Like you didn't enjoy all the sex as much as I did? The guy who counted the times he came in one night and measured the length of his cock with a ruler? So, you were just putting up with the sex to have someone to watch *Law and Order* with on the hotel TV and talk about social injustice and share a midnight pizza after the burden of sex?

Him: Of course, I enjoyed all the fooling around. I know you know that. But I need more than that. I told you early on that I get bored easily.

Me: Well, if you got bored with me, that I could understand. But don't say I treated you like a whore.

Him: I wasn't bored with you. I was bored with the dynamic. Trying to talk to you was getting more and more impossible. You would shut down. You know that's true.

Me: You're right. I would. Trying to justify my beliefs was a chore, and I didn't feel safe opening up to you about what I really thought.

Him: AHA! So, you treated me like a whore.

Me: This is getting us nowhere. I am done.

The words said that day would haunt me for months. Hank's heretofore withheld nasty judgments flew from his fingertips like lasers to my heart. I wanted to vomit—to purge his words, his sentiments—all of him—from my body and my memory. But that's not how it works. How do you erase part of your life? You can't. At least, I couldn't. I had always taken what people said to me seriously. Words had import. Maybe it was an occupational hazard.

So I asked myself whether this was true. I asked my husband and my metamour and my friends, "Did I treat Hank like a whore? If not, then why would Hank say this to me? He wouldn't hurt me for sport, right?"

Eric said, "No. You treated him well. Sometimes, people say hurtful things to make the breakup easier."

Marianne said, "No. That was inexcusable behavior on his part."

My close girlfriends said the same. Trisha knew Hank from the time the three of us and Hank's buddy had played pool one Saturday night. She said, "Honey, trust me, it's not true. I've seen how he looked at you and acted with you. I'm so sorry he said those things. You may not want to hear this, but I think you are better off."

Their supportive and well-meaning explanations had little effect on me compared to the missives from Hank. I read them over and over and over, obsessively hunting for answers, as if the solution was in code, if only I were smart enough to decipher it.

The effect of my breakup splashed onto Eric. He had started casually seeing a young woman named Zella, in addition to being in the second year of his long-term relationship with Marianne. Zella worked a retail job blocks from our house and napped on our sofa during split shifts to save her the hour-long drive home. I was embarrassed when I learned that Eric told Zella, "Natalie is raw from a recent breakup with her boyfriend, so tread lightly." A quiet and creative girl with a poet's soul, she offered home-baked goods as gratitude and did indeed tread lightly—so lightly that I thought of her more as a family friend than as a metamour. Maybe I was too distracted by my own relationship postmortem to devote much attention to Eric's dating life, which I saw as gliding on greased rails while mine crashed on broken tracks.

Hank was my first real breakup of consequence. His parting shots made me question our whole relationship, but as I reexamined every encounter, I could not agree that I treated him poorly.

* * *

The Hank and Sylvia saga lasted four years. I dated Hank for two, we did not see each other for another year, we tried to be friends and maybe more, but there was more conflict. Then we didn't see each other for another year, and then we did, and it was nice for a very brief time, and then it wasn't.

I finally gave up, exhausted. I had no more affection and support to give. I felt he had lied to me about his other relationships, my place in his life, and his intentions.

I learned that honesty is hard for some people, but that polyamory—my polyamory—required it. I am not sure I got any better at detecting bullshit, but I became more prepared for it when I discovered I had stepped in it.

Polyamory had led me here. I had exposed myself to emotional carnage when I was married to a man who did not say things to wound me. I was kidding myself that an actual long-term polyamorous relationship outside my marriage would work for me. Maybe it worked for Eric, but for me, hookups and casual sex were all I could expect. I wondered whether all secondary or "other" poly relationships were inherently temporary.

In an effort to start fresh and encourage positive karma, I turned the page to the new calendar year by wishing Hank a happy one. I disliked holding grudges. It took too much energy.

15.

Metamour with a Teramour

Leah offered a new twist. She was unmarried and lived with her primary partner, Ronan. Eric was not her sole means of emotional support and physical play.

Eric made a point to regularly check in with Leah and with his new metamour about Eric and Leah's relationship. I was called upon only periodically for metamour and teramour maintenance. *Teramour* was a term our polycule came to use (shout out to Violet) for a metamour's non-shared partner. Other poly folks use the term *telemour*, broadly meaning distant love. To foster connection, the four of us spent time together over grilled steaks and movie outings.

After Marianne moved to monogamy land, Leah filled the girlfriend gap, and I was grateful for her. That Eric had an enthusiastic partner for kink and swinger activities alleviated my guilt. Plus, I got to experience compersion, that heart-filling happiness at seeing your partner happy with another partner.

While dating Leah, Eric started attending a 10,000-person camping event in northwestern Pennsylvania called Pennsic, that Leah and Ronan had attended. It was an annual burner-meets-renaissance festival with classes in medieval arts such as palmistry, astronomy, fire-starting, and history and participation in live action role-playing (LARPing) as knights, royalty, warriors, peasants, and performers.

Eric embraced the lazy afternoons of drinking from a tankard, socializing, drumming around a campfire, or napping in a hammock alone or with Leah. He enjoyed the quirky and hedonistic people, some of whom traveled across the country with their families, friends, lovers, or alone. He reveled in the naked spaghetti parties and took notes at the sundial-making classes. He drank up the atmosphere with a king-sized goblet. Bless his heart, he wanted to share his wondrous experience with me, but I was not a camper. The beach was more my jam.

Leah loved Pennsic-ing with both her partners, sleeping with each one on alternating nights when both Eric and Ronan attended. Thanks to polyamory, I could spend guilt-free time at home—and partake of air conditioning!—after traveling for work twice the prior month, and Eric would have a partner in medieval fun and stories to share with me on his return.

The year Ronan couldn't attend Pennsic due to work, I found a handwritten card in the mailbox the day after Leah and Eric left for Pennsylvania.

> Hi Natalie,
>
> Thank you for letting me borrow your husband for two weeks. I love to go camping and to events like this, and it's much more fulfilling when I have someone to share the experience with. I think you would have a wonderful time here as well, but I am biased.
>
> I hope you're having a wonderful time as well. Ronan told me he gave you a pool pass for our place, so you're welcome to enjoy it whenever. It's open until 10 at night! I like swimming under the stars.
>
> I will do my best to return your husband in one piece.
>
> You know how he is, though, so no promises.
>
> XOXO
> Leah

I felt fortunate to have Leah in our lives, not only because she was a positive, unconventional, free-spirited person (my foil, perhaps), but because she filled needs in Eric that I did not. Leah was tall, her hair dyed in an ever-changing swirl of colors from teal to watermelon. She spent hours transforming herself with makeup, platform shoes, and her sewing creations in preparation for artistic performances. On one night, she danced with swords and balloons, and on another, she smeared herself with fake blood while writhing to dark music. Eric, very often in attendance with his metamour, Ronan, would cheer her on. After I saw her perform, I hugged her close in support, risking a sprinkling of her turquoise glitter eye shadow. I admired her style.

When Eric proposed an outing that I found myself wincing at, I was grateful to be able to say, "I appreciate that you want to spend time with me and share in this experience, but that sounds like something Leah would like." Sometimes, the three or four of us did hang out together. When Leah, Eric, and I went to a Gwar concert, an over-the-top metal performance band from Richmond that Leah had been dying to see, she was belly to the stage and got the fan girl experience. We both got a kick out of her full-throttle enjoyment, and we all left the show exhilarated and exhausted, dropping Leah at home where Ronan was waiting to hear all about it.

Ronan cherished Leah. He would see a furry cat-shaped magenta handbag and think, "Leah would like that," and buy it for her. He randomly brought home flowers and sweets if she was having a rough week. I had never seen anyone so spoiled for her birthday. One year, Ronan planned a party at a swanky restaurant with a dozen friends, and he and Eric gave her a custom-made belly-dancing outfit. I baked her a graveyard cake topped with a three-dimensional tapered hexagonal coffin I fashioned out of chocolate. Her squeals of delight echoed in a roomful of polyamorists.

As much as I liked Leah, at times I struggled with the voice in my head that told me I was not enough of something that my metamour was. I was not bisexual. I couldn't pole dance. I didn't surprise Eric with a different hue of hair color every month or two. No one ever paid me to model for a fetish magazine or to eat messy foods on camera. I have never shed my top at a rock concert and tossed my bra on stage, to Eric's delight. I was not a childless thirtysomething, and even if I were, I would not have had the guts to do half the things Leah did or wear half the skimpy and amazing wardrobe pieces she created and inhabited with easy confidence.

It was not so much that I wished I were younger or could swing a hula hoop on my hips like Leah could, but when I saw how much Eric enjoyed that about her, I felt less. Eric rolled his eyes at my insecurities, but he also pulled me onto his lap and put his arms around me as tears welled up in my eyes.

"Yes," he said. "I do love all those things about Leah. I am lucky to have both of you in my life. I don't want you to be like Leah, and I don't want Leah to be like you."

He reminded my fragile, middle-aged ego of all the things he loved about me, such as how he couldn't keep his hands off my sexy curves, and how he would be lost without my competence and partnership. He grinned as he told me that he loved how I drop everything to dance barefoot with him to "Life in the Fast Lane" under the strobe light he affixed to the living room ceiling. He derived joy from seeing me beam with schoolgirl wonder at the colored spots of light jumping off the carpet and the wall, and dancing reminds him of the long-haired, studious but sultry coed he fell in love with.

After a few minutes of self-indulgent cuddling and reassurances I'm embarrassed to admit I need, I felt better. I felt grounded. I loved all those things about Leah as well. I also loved all those other things about myself. I'm a great catch, and I was grateful that Eric cherished me for who I am. He showed how he felt about me every day by waking up beside me, parenting with me, scratching that spot on my back I couldn't reach, and kissing me in a way that still makes me blush.

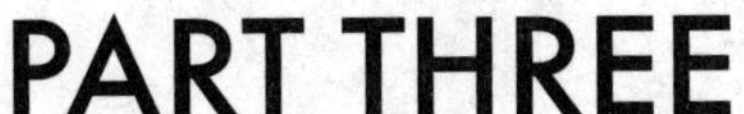

PART THREE

16.

Recovery

On a spring evening, I was filling time at the Orlando airport while I waited to fly back to DC. I scrolled through old messages from OkCupid, the dating site I used in the year and a half I had been dating Hank. Most of my experiences on the site were mediocre one-offs. Some dates led to recurring intimacies with polyamorous men who traveled to DC for work. I was still new to poly dating, and I wanted to see what was out there, as Hank knew. I didn't message Hank in the evenings. That was his family time.

Lee's profile photos caught my attention. In one, he was holding a baby as he stood on the steps of the Supreme Court. The caption read, "Someday, my daughter is going to preside there as Chief Justice." In the other photo, he mowed the lawn while wearing a child's fireman hat. I imagined his daughter had perched it on his head with a giggle, and his wife, catching him in the act, had snapped a photo.

I sat on a stiff plastic airport chair, still in my business suit and heels. After a long workday and challenges with Hank a year and a half into our relationship, Lee seemed like a good guy, but I was in a mood that dared him to tell me to fuck off.

Sighing to myself that he lived at least thirty minutes from me—the same distance as Hank—I messaged him, "I think that your location makes you logistically undesirable, but maybe not?"

His profile told me he was a polyamorous married dad and liked to make ice cream and watch baseball. The married status made me pause because of the turbulence with Sylvia, but I tried not to judge a new relationship by the sins of the prior ones, my sins included.

Lee didn't tell me to fuck off. He seemed mildly amused by my ramblings and suggested we get a drink. I thought, *What the hell. I haven't scared him off yet.*

Our first date was on a Sunday. Eric pretended to be wounded that I was meeting another guy on our wedding anniversary. We didn't make a big deal out of such annual markers; we had spent a quiet dinner together the night before and exchanged cards that morning.

Lee was sitting at the bar when I arrived. When he stood, I could see he was over six feet tall and lean with short hair. From his online photos, I recognized the plaid, Western-style shirt with snaps.

He greeted me with a warm smile that overtook his face. At his suggestion, we moved to a table in a dark corner. The bar was almost empty on a Sunday evening. Our getting-acquainted conversation was easy. I felt a mutual attraction, so when he sidled next to me, grinned, and said that he was going to kiss me because we should "get this over with," I was grateful. There was no reason to draw out the question of whether we had chemistry. Attraction mattered.

I appreciated not having to take the lead. There had been times at the end of a date when the guy was so awkward about "closing the deal," as Hank would say, that I took the initiative and kissed him because I needed to know. I didn't want to wait three dates for him to get up his nerve.

I knew women who took a few dates to warm up, to evaluate, to decide. I was not that woman. Every time I ignored my instincts because the guy was nice and looked good on paper, and we had a pleasant but not electric time, the relationship would limp along, with me hoping the attraction would grow. It never did.

Ending a three-month relationship was harder than saying after the first date, "It was nice meeting you, but I am not feeling the connection I am looking for." I found that when I spoke up after the first date, guys appreciated the honesty. No one liked to be strung along or ghosted.

After kissing Lee in the bar, followed by more extended making out in his car, we both felt the heat and started dating.

Early in my relationship with Lee, I had driven to his house after his daughter was in bed. His wife, Winnie, was on a date. Lee and I had fun getting to know each other better in and out of the bedroom. As I was preparing to leave, Winnie texted Lee that she was on her way home.

"I know it's getting late, but do you mind staying a little longer to meet Winnie?"

I was anxious about meeting Lee's wife. My confidence in being a good metamour had drained slowly, succubus-style, after a year and a half with Sylvia.

But I had to meet her sometime. I screwed up my courage.

"I can stay a bit," I said.

Lee and I were sitting on the living room couch when Winnie walked in the front door. We both stood up. Lee walked to the entryway and gave his wife a welcome home kiss. I thought, *How sweet.* I had never witnessed that simple tenderness between Sylvia and Hank.

After they disengaged, I slowly approached Winnie, trying to remember how my limbs operated. I braced myself for a scowl, a judging once-over, or, if I was lucky, maybe just indifference. I may have micro-flinched.

"Winnie, this is Nat," Lee said.

Winnie's eyes met mine. Her face lit up in a smile. Then she drew me into a full-body hug, vibrating with warmth.

"I am so happy to meet you!" she said.

I felt as if a valve had opened at the top of my head. The tension rose out of my scalp like steam and dissipated. I will remember her smile forever. I could hear the universe saying, *Hey, girl, we know things were challenging with Sylvia, but polyamory is not always like that. Hang in there.*

Winnie plopped down on the loveseat, positioned at a right angle to the couch. I carefully lowered myself onto the couch next to Lee. Winnie talked easily about her evening, a first date, in a self-deprecating but self-assured manner, laughing about her clumsiness during the date, showing us the wine splashes on her top. Winnie radiated compersion that her husband had found someone he connected with, and she wanted to get to know that someone. At least that's how she seemed to me. Maybe I was so relieved at her friendliness that all I could see were unicorns prancing over rainbows.

I was mindful not to sit too close to Lee, although I doubt it would have fazed Winnie if I had sat on his lap. I think my Sylvia scar tissue was trying to protect me from offending her.

We three interacted with refreshing ease, talking and laughing about first dates. I stayed later than I had anticipated and left feeling accepted, as if I had been granted a cosmic do-over.

I carried this positive feeling with me on my drive home. I pictured Winnie asking Lee about our evening and listening to any details he wanted to share, with interest and love. That thought made me feel connected philosophically because that was how Eric would be with me after a date. Seeing Winnie and Lee interact gave me comfort that their relationship was healthy enough to support my entering the picture. At the very least, I didn't feel a negative vibe.

Over the coming weeks and months, I found Lee to be a refreshing blend of fully formed adult, responsible parent, and attentive husband. He was also a geeky, adventuresome, tender guy with a bit of the overgrown adolescent in him. He said "I'm in!" to my invitation to an Oz-themed dance party at a fetish club. He dressed like the Tin Man, aided by his wife's style sense. Winnie had helped him fashion an oil can cap, spray-painted silver. With his lanky frame, he fit the part to a T. My closet was devoid of blue and white gingham, so I opted to embrace the club vibe by wearing a black latex bra top and a black latex skirt with red piping, shined to a seal-like sleekness. In the back room of the sex-positive club, I discovered that Lee was game for some naughtiness as he snaked his hand up my clinging skirt while I perched on a bar stool, standing on its lower metal ring to match his height as I moaned against his chest.

Lee shared an erotic story he wrote about our first time together in a hotel, making me blush at his graphic boldness so early in our relationship. He was also up for stealing some passion in his office suite after hours, enjoying dinner and a movie, getting a hotel room, or even staying overnight at my place without having to creep home at 2:00 a.m.

Will's room was on the same floor as our master bedroom. The extra bedroom in our house was on the top floor. When Eric and I both had guests on the same night, I typically took the master, and Eric took the room overhead.

One night, when Lee came home with me, the teen's door was shut. I assumed he was asleep or gaming with his headphones on. Eric was on the top floor with Marianne. Lee and I were deep into each other, and I lost myself in the heat of the moment. The next thing I knew, there was a voice outside my bedroom door.

"Mom, are you okay?"

Sproinggg!

Lee sprang out of the bed like a cartoon character. He stage-whispered, "Where should I go? Bathroom or closet?"

I stifled a laugh at Lee's naked frame, ready to dart as instructed. Shrugging, I answered, "Closet?" I pulled on my robe and opened the locked bedroom door.

"I'm fine, honey. Just a bad dream," I said.

His furrowed brow relaxed, and he padded back to his room. I closed my door.

Lee emerged from his hiding place. I was caught between laughter and apologies. Lee complimented me on how organized my closet was. I blushed, picturing my label-maker-tagged storage bin for FISHNETS.

I wondered if Lee would grab his clothes and say, "That was too close. I'm out of here," but he didn't.

He slid back into bed and said, "Okay, c'mon, Will must know what's up, right?"

"No, trust me. He's in his own world. He likes it there."

After Lee shook off the interruption, we managed to pick up where we left off.

The next morning, Will slept late like a typical teenager. Eric and Marianne started the coffee. Lee made chocolate chip pancakes. I scrambled eggs. When Will lumbered down the stairs, rubbing sleep from his eyes, we four adults were finishing breakfast and watching a silly video on the laptop.

"Lee made pancakes," I said. "They're on the counter if you want some."

Will was used to seeing Marianne at weekend breakfast, but that was the first time there had been a fourth addition to our brunch crew. He was unfazed or, more likely, disinterested. If a monkey had been perched on the kitchen counter washing dishes, Will might well have handed over his plate and returned to his teen cave.

Not only could Lee stay over and enjoy breakfast with my family, but I was allowed to sleep at his house and interact with his daughter and his wife. Having Winnie was a game-changer after the trial by fire with Sylvia.

Winnie and Lee hosted a poly barbecue a month after Lee and I started dating. Eric invited Marianne, who was happy to join us. Hank and Sylvia did not attend despite my invitation. At the poly-cue, Lee, the grill master, introduced us to everyone as they arrived. I met Winnie and Lee's adorable preschooler, their other lovers, their friends, and other poly folks. Winnie's guests included her girlfriend, her girlfriend's primary partner, and their child, as well as a single guy Winnie was dating.

My contribution to the cookout was a cake I baked in a pan that Sylvia had given to me as one of her apology gifts, and I felt she was with me in spirit at the party. I was glowing with poly positivity.

Dating half of a married couple that was outwardly comfortable with polyamory was a new dynamic for me. Winnie and Lee were both dating, and from what I could see, they were in love and happy together, in stark contrast to Sylvia's sniping and Hank's grumbling. Lee and Winnie's interactions with each other and their daughter comforted me. I dared myself to hope that chaos and unpredictability were not the cornerstones of polyamory.

Over the subsequent months, I found myself wanting to know Winnie better. She exuded kindness. Smart and savvy, she was someone I would have wanted as a friend, with or without her husband as our V. Only three years younger than me, she was much closer to my age than my prior metamours.

I never thought Winnie was trying to undermine my relationship with Lee, that she had a secret agenda, or that she was struggling with polyamory. I didn't have to bring her along the poly path, take baby steps, or bend over backward and watch every word I said or action I took. The liberation was intoxicating.

Winnie and I began to develop a friendship. She invited me to her ritzy new fitness club. Unlike my no-frills neighborhood Gold's Gym, where I attended low-tech step aerobics classes and got a few miles in on the cardio machines, Winnie's club boasted a swimming pool, a sauna, and multiple jacuzzi tubs. I accepted one of her guest passes for a Saturday metamour outing.

As many moms know, the gym can be a sacred space. No one is asking us for anything. The only folks pushing us are ourselves. No matter how many dozen people are sweating elbow-to-elbow with me, I could be as alone as I wanted to be, with my music thumping through my earbuds to spur me on as I rowed, or an audiobook sweet-talking me on the elliptical. It was my time.

Winnie had raved about Reformer Pilates, so although I was skeptical of a workout that involved planks, springs, and pulleys that called to mind a medieval torture device, I gave it a go. I was delighted when it unkinked my back and worked my core. I exercised muscles I suspected would ache the next day, but ache in a good way. After a relaxed conversation over salads and smoothies at the club café, we headed to the locker room to unwind in the whirlpool.

As we undressed, I recalled Lee comparing my body to Winnie's in the essay he had written about our first sexual encounter. Reading it before meeting Winnie, I had bristled at the comparison, as if a third party had been present in our hotel room. In the locker room, when I noted in passing the similarities in our shapes, I saw what Lee had seen. I felt a stronger connection to Winnie, as if Lee's appreciation of our bodies' commonalities, as well as their differences, made us more kindred.

My interactions with Winnie helped me feel that polyamory was fitting me better, like trying on jeans you finally feel comfortable in. Even so, part of me was still internally negotiating, weighing, waiting for the seam to split from an unseen, careless stitch. Damn if I would let myself fall into a metamour sinkhole because I wanted success so badly. My eyes might have been clouded with affection for my metamour, but they were still open.

In the spa, we luxuriated in the heat and bubbles, away from kids and husbands, chores and obligations. We talked about the things that new friends talk about—family, relationships, favorite movies, whether language immersion schools were a good idea, where we were in our careers and where we wanted to go, and the various curses of the female body, including the quest for bras that fit. Winnie, thankfully, took the lead.

She told me about her prior marriage and how she met Lee, who was single and ten years her junior. She had thought that Lee would be a fun distraction after she and her husband opened up their marriage. She had told her husband as much at the time, saying, "There's a cute guy at the office. I think I will have a little fling with him." She recounted to me their working together, hooking up with feverish intensity wherever and whenever they could, in office closets, cars, the rare motel room, and falling in love.

When they realized that theirs was not a casual affair, Lee broke up with his longtime girlfriend, and Winnie and her husband separated. I cannot remember what I shared with her, but I suspect it was far less. I may have told her that my dating history was barely a blip before I married Eric and about our foray into swinging and then into polyamory. I probably told her some more about Hank and Sylvia, depending on the drama of the day, since I was still seeing Hank at that time.

I didn't get the sense that Winnie was sharing her history to warn me off or to impress me, but rather that she was simply telling her story. It was a story about a man we shared. I appreciated the insight into Lee and her.

While I hoped for a positive poly relationship experience with Lee and his partners, I also needed my connection with Lee to include an intense physical component. Dating Hank had loosed a daring side that I wanted to keep alive, and Lee was game for my explorations. When you're married with kids and dating someone married with kids, sometimes you need to be creative.

On the evening that I treated Lee to a birthday dinner, we arrived at a dining experience evocative of Moulin Rouge, hiding in plain sight. The interior of a staid downtown office building had been remodeled. From the beige stone exterior, you would never know that inside, it was two stories, open-loft style, complete with a glass-enclosed stage for the cabaret on the second floor. Mardi Gras mask-wearing waitstaff offered slender halogen lamps to help patrons read the menus at the low-lit tables.

The restaurant was adorned with burgundy velvet draperies and burlesque-inspired murals satirizing politics and culture. One wall was painted with the image of an almost nude former president playing saxophone. An ebony-haired, fleshy young woman clad in a scanty toga held his waist as they perched atop a white stallion, their full heads of hair swaying, as if in motion.

The vibe led me to imagine salacious goings-on in a private back room for those who knew the code phrase—"The raven caws at midnight"—or perhaps those who possessed an ivory-colored calling card, embossed in gothic script with the password "Nevermore."

Our table was on the second floor, affording us a direct view of the stage. We ordered wine and appetizers we could share, including a decadent fondue. We fed the skewered, cheese-coated bread cubes to ourselves and, more messily, to each other.

As we finished our meal, Cirque du Soleil–type performers in lingerie and dramatic makeup athletically contorted their fit bodies in time with the piped-in music. The show was a steamy aphrodisiac. Lee's hand reached under the table and rested on my thigh, bare above my leather boot. I pressed my thighs together, trapping his hand for a moment, locking his eyes to mine.

"Shall we get the check?" asked Lee. I nodded.

It was too early to go to my house since Will would still be awake. Lee's house was too far away. Downtown hotels were pricey.

"We can walk to my office if you don't mind the cold," Lee suggested.

"I'm game." I smiled up at him. I thought a brisk walk in the cool night, after a heavy meal and heady entertainment, might tamp the flush of warmth I felt and halt me igniting from within. Lee's hand in mine, however, deliciously frustrated that goal.

Lee worked in an office suite in a multi-storied building. Window offices and meeting rooms lined the perimeter. The interior held open cubicles, lounge areas, small offices with doors, and a kitchen. I had tasted Nutella for the first time in that kitchen some weeks before. Our last sexcapade had been on the long conference room table where Lee attended weekly meetings. We had been in search of a post-shagging snack. I had concluded that Nutella needed an FDA warning label: "CAUTION: Be advised that a single serving may lead to addiction." Since then, I have avoided open jars of the stuff as I would packets of heroin.

This time, Lee dropped his backpack on one of the sofas. All was quiet. I didn't know the full layout of the suite, but it was larger than I thought. I was feeling mischievous.

"Give me a half-minute lead," I said.

Lee's left eyebrow rose, and a bemused grin played upon his lips.

"Okay," he said.

I turned a corner and paused to unzip one calf-high boot, then the other, dropping them in my wake. I skipped across an open area in socks and shrugged off my wool coat, letting it fall to the floor. At the next turn, off came my scarlet scarf, landing on the carpet like a twisted smile.

I was a little out of breath, but I didn't want Lee to catch up before my plan was fully hatched. The adrenaline of the chase was upon me.

I came to an interior office and ventured inside. The room was no more than eight by eight feet. It held a desk facing the door and a chair near the door. There was nothing else in the room, not even a phone or a trash can. I placed my bag outside the door and went back inside the tiny office, leaving the door ajar.

I climbed onto the desk, shifting positions to what I hoped was an alluring, semi-reclining, centerfold pose. Lying on the desk, I rested my head in my cupped palm and cocked my hip. My heart was beating wildly, and my face was flushed. I felt somewhat silly, but I pushed that thought aside.

Fortunately, Lee was not far behind, or I likely would have lost my nerve. He slowly pushed open the door, his hands full of my discarded clothes.

"I think I found everything." He laughed and placed my belongings in a corner.

Lee joined me on top of the desk. His lips brushed the side of my neck and down into the space where my sweater dipped. I pulled it over my head and tossed it with my other clothes.

He was a long, angular six-foot-four, and making out on the desk, while steamy, became awkward.

"Lie down," he said. He gently nudged me onto my back, cupping my head to save it from banging the desk.

"Move up a bit," he said.

I shimmied up. I still had on my bra, panties, skirt, and socks. Lee pulled off my panties.

"Stay there, please," he said.

He moved the lone chair to the end of the desk by my feet. He pushed up my skirt past my hips and settled into the chair. His hands, and then his face, were under my skirt. I began to squirm. Low moans escaped me.

My head rested on one end of the hard desk. Lee's face was at the other. As I was enjoying the moment, I turned my face toward the door. Through the narrow backlit window running down the side of the door, I saw a shadow. It got larger, filling the window frame, and then withdrew suddenly. I could barely make out a female face with lips formed in an "oh."

I tried unsuccessfully to stifle a laugh.

"Lee," I whispered. He did not respond. His mouth was occupied.

"Lee," I whispered more loudly. "I think the cleaning woman just looked in through that window."

He bolted upright.

"Shit," he said, scrambling.

"Oh, please don't stop. I was so close," I teased.

"Natalie, I work here! I left my backpack out there. I have to go out there and get my stuff."

Lee, typically laid back, was much less amused than I was.

He cracked the door an inch and peered out as if we were in a wacky rom-com caper movie and the bad guys were looking for us.

"I'll go out first. You get dressed." He darted out. I was impressed with his agility. I could not help but chuckle.

It took me a moment to find my sweater, and I pulled it over my head. I buttoned my coat, picked up my scarf, and slung my bag over my shoulder. I poked my head out, as Lee had just done, and I laughed again. The coast was clear. That was good, I guessed. I retraced my steps to where we had entered the office suite and saw Lee. He was bouncing from one foot to the other, antsy to leave the premises.

"Did you see the cleaning woman?" I asked.

"No, she must have gone to another floor. Let's get out of here before she comes back."

That was the last time Lee and I were in his office. He changed jobs soon after the Cleaning Woman Incident. I will never forget the cleaner's shocked expression, nor Lee's instinctive fight or flight response. I pondered my initiative, and then my giggly reaction at being spotted in a compromising position. It surprised me that I was not embarrassed or ashamed of having sex in an office, and with a man who was not my husband. I was amused, even thrilled, at being caught in the act. How naughty.

Polyamory had brought out a side of me I had not known I had. It was a side that did not belong to the straight A, straitlaced, snarky, somewhat self-conscious girl I had been, or considered myself to be. I wondered if polyamory had created this woman out of whole cloth, or if it had merely given her the opportunity—and permission—to emerge.

* * *

Lee worked for a progressive organization. Soon after we started dating, he attended a team-building office retreat, complete with sharing and bonding and drinking.

One session addressed discrimination in the workplace, including the ability to be your truest and best self at work. Some of Lee's colleagues shared how their beliefs, sexual orientation, gender, or other identity exposed them to prejudice on the job. Lee, in turn, expressed his concern about the repercussions of being honest about his relationship lifestyle. He told the assembled group that he and his wife were in an open marriage because polyamory was part of his identity.

Picture applause from his colleagues for his courage and transparency and shouts of support, subdued nods, or reassuring pats on the arm. Imagine the discussion that was spurred about what it was like to be a minority in the workplace because of how and who you love.

But Lee heard only the buzz of the air conditioner. At the next session break, his coworkers acted as if that moment had been sucked into a time vortex, as if he had not told them he was polyamorous.

Some months later, a coworker good-naturedly goaded him about wearing a tie at their casual office. My lover smiled and said his girlfriend—that would be me—was taking him out for a fancy birthday dinner. Lee's response was met not with willful deafness, but with physical retreat, as the colleague backed away. When he told me this story, I could tell how it hurt him that his friends and colleagues refused to see him.

Once his colleagues had been told, they were stuck with the knowledge and any accompanying personal discomfort. They dealt with it by pretending they did not know it. Maybe it was like avoiding the unease of eye contact with someone in a wheelchair when we all just want to be seen.

So many times, I wished my work friends knew I was polyamorous. It would have made talking about my weekend easier. I spent a lot of time with unnamed friends for weekend bike rides, hiking, or eating out. Everyone at my office knew I was married, but no one asked for details. Perhaps I gave them too little credit, and everyone knew I was a poly slut but simply shrugged.

When adultery, open marriages, and related topics came up at the office, I wanted to step onto my poly soapbox and reference my lived experience, but I could only skirt the edges. When an officemate sniggered about someone in an open marriage, I said, "I have heard of that being an option when everyone is honest about what they want." When my colleague said, "Natalie, would you date some younger guy?" I said, "Sure, why not—who would I be hurting?"

An officemate who taught Sunday school at a Unitarian fellowship told our coffee klatch that he had invited a lesbian guest speaker to talk to his class about polyamory. I said, "That's great that you are exposing the kids to orientation, lifestyle, and relationship options!" I wanted to say much more.

When office chat turned to the most recent politician to get caught with his pants down, I suggested that maybe he should have been honest with his wife. Then she could have explored an extramarital relationship, too. What I did not say at the time was "I know what I am talking about, guys, because that's my life. That's the life Eric and I share. We don't lie or cheat. We have a full physical and emotional relationship with each other *and* make connections with others. I highly recommend it." But I recalled the reactions of Lee's colleagues and held my tongue.

To be fair, not everyone at Lee's office had a negative reaction. One young colleague asked him more about his relationship dynamic, an interaction Lee embraced. By taking a personal risk, Lee had moved the conversation forward to normalizing non-monogamy. I admired him.

I was not that brave. It was quite possible that some of my colleagues, most of whom I respected as rational, thoughtful people, would have been supportive, respectfully inquisitive, or at least kept their judgments to themselves. I thought

I would come out to them at some point—either on my last day of work or after too much alcohol.

* * *

Lee tried to coordinate our dates with his wife's dating schedule. While a considerate practice in general to avoid one partner feeling left out, this was a necessity for them because they could not leave their daughter alone. One parent stayed home while the other was out.

I had been dating Lee for a few months, and we were having a post-sex snack at the kitchen table when Winnie came home from a date. We all exchanged hugs. Winnie pulled up a chair to tell us about her evening.

I complimented Winnie on her outfit. She said that she was wearing flats because her date was not tall. As one is wont to do after a first date, she was processing out loud. He reminded her of an actor we were familiar with. He was in finance, as Winnie had been some years ago. She found him attractive, witty, and fun and thought she would like to see him again. Lee and I were happy to hear that her date had gone well. I drove home, kissed Eric, and got ready for bed. It was a weeknight, so my schedule for the next day was percolating in my head—getting Will to school, work, and after-work obligations.

The next morning, I stood in my closet, considering what to wear. I had a drinks date with someone new at a restaurant a few blocks from my office, so I wanted to wear an outfit that transitioned easily between work and play. I chose a clingier top and a shorter skirt than if I had meetings or a court appearance.

It was autumn, World Series time. Lee and Winnie were rooting for opposite teams from their respective hometowns. There was also a strange beard phenomenon occurring. Presumably due to superstition, a player for one of the teams said he would not shave while the Series was ongoing. His teammates took up his cause, and beards sprouted everywhere. I didn't like beards. They got in the way. When fans started growing beards in support, I wondered if Schick and Gillette stock went down.

After work, I walked to the meetup spot. My online name was a pseudonym. I often did not tell my date my real name until right before we met. I might text it or just introduce myself when we met. My date had told me his first name in a private message. Maybe I was overly cautious, but no one complained.

The restaurant where I met my date had been the scene of several of my first dates. It was an easy walk from my office, but not so close or popular that my officemates would be there. I could usually find two empty bar stools together, and the happy hour prices were good. They served small plates, which were convenient for nibbling without committing to dinner. I wondered what the bartenders thought, if anything, about my repeat visits, each time with a different guy, and if they heard us talking about *poly*, *open relationship*, or *my husband's girlfriend*.

My date was sitting at the bar. I thought I recognized him from the online photos he posted and from his description of what he would be wearing. Mainly, I recognized the expression of someone waiting for someone. He was clean-shaven in his profile photo, but like every third guy in town, he was sporting the World Series beard. He was from the town where one of the teams played.

My first thought was *damn beards*. Even Lee had stopped shaving to prove to Winnie—who liked beards—that he was incapable of growing a decent one. When I had looked askance at Lee's scraggly facial hair, he told me that his scruff would go the way of flip phones after the Series ended.

We ordered drinks, red wine for me and a beer for my date. We chatted about typical first-date things, like where we were from, our families, travel, and our work. He was single and new to polyamory, so I filled him in on my situation and the mechanics of open relationships.

"I'm married," I said, "as I am sure you saw in my dating profile. I'm also currently seeing a guy who is married with a young daughter."

"Yeah, I saw that," he said, his eyes darting to the TV over the bar that was airing the warmup to the baseball game. "I hope you don't mind, but I want to leave in time to catch the game at home."

"That's cool," I said, shrugging. "The guy I'm dating, Lee, and his wife, Winnie, are rooting for opposite teams. I have my fingers crossed that the marital strife is minimal. I like him *and* his wife, and don't want to get in the middle of sports drama," I joked.

I was on my second glass of wine and feeling the alcohol on my empty stomach. I was not sure if it was the expression on my date's face as I talked about Winnie and her family, including their adorable kid, or that my synapses started firing on all cylinders, but I looked at him more closely. He was not tall, and as I focused on him, I saw that he bore some resemblance to an actor I was familiar with. What did he say he did for work? Oh, yes, he was in finance, with an office down the street from Lee's.

I stopped talking and swiveled left on my bar stool to face him squarely.

"Did you have a date last night?" I asked.

"Yes," he said. Was that a slight twinkle in his eye?

"Was her name Winnie?" I asked.

"Yes." He smirked. I smiled.

"Were you going to tell me?" I asked.

"Maybe?" he half-asked and half-stated, with raised eyebrows and an uncertain grin.

I threw my head back and laughed. I had caught him, poor not-poly guy, who had the dumb luck to date, on two consecutive nights, the two arms of the same polyamorous V. What were the odds? I could not bring myself to fault him for being a deer caught in headlights when it became clear, as it must have when I started talking about the woman he had met the previous night, and both she and I had mentioned each other *by name* to him. Chalk up another poly first for me. I didn't know the protocol for him or for me.

Through my laughter and slight alcohol haze, I gushed, "Winnie is so awesome. Do you think you'll see her again?"

He said, "Maybe."

Even though he could have come clean before being confronted, I was more amused than anything.

"Is this small poly world freaking you out? It's hilarious to me."

"Not really," he said, "but I'm not sure."

"Fair enough," I said.

At the bar, we kissed goodbye, and he went home to watch the game. I stayed and finished my wine, smiling as I shook my head and snickered some more. I found it comforting to experience how interconnected we all were.

The next day, I sent a message to Winnie. "Guess who I had drinks with last night?" Multiple texting acronyms and emoticons for laughter and incredulity ensued.

I asked Winnie, "Do you think you'll see him again?"

"Yes, I think so," she replied. "Are you okay with that?"

"Sure! He's attractive, smart, and fun to be with. Go for it," I replied.

"Do you think you would see him again?" she asked.

"Hmm, I don't know," I responded. "I wouldn't rule it out."

We agreed to see how it shook out and that we were cool with whatever happened.

Lee, however, was feeling weird at the thought of both the women he was sleeping with potentially dating the same guy. He said it was more about sharing limited resources than anything.

The new guy seemed fine with it all, at least fine enough that he asked us both out again.

After my second date with him, I decided not to have a third. He was nice enough, but I did not feel the spark. I was never a pogonophile—lover of beards—as a more extended kiss on the second date confirmed.

Practically speaking, I was more jazzed for Winnie to have a new relationship, as was Lee, not only because we were happy for her, but also because then she would be having her own fun while Lee and I were having ours. As a polyamorist, I strove to be cognizant of the needs of my partners and metamours. They affected me. If, for example, I had a date on a night when Eric's plans fell through, I felt some guilt. Eric never placed that guilt on me, but I felt it. So too, Eric might wait and see how my weekly plans were shaping up before confirming his. This derived from common courtesy and feelings of compersion which extended to my metamours, especially those I connected with like Winnie.

When I considered who I would rather spend time with, it was Lee, not Winnie's potential new beau. Nor did I relish competing with Winnie for time with not just Lee, but the new guy. They say polyamorists spend more time scheduling than having sex, and I wanted less of the former and more of the latter. Polyamory teaches the value and limits of time. Who did I want to spend time with when time was limited? Speaking of the limits of time, Winnie's new relationship only lasted a month or two until scheduling logistics and driving distances got the best of them.

Winnie's and my peacefully coexisting as arms of a bearded V made me realize how far I had come from the default of jealousy inherent in many monogamous dynamics. As a polyamorist, I experienced compersion for my metamour. Granted, if we had both continued to date the new guy, I could not say for certain what the impact on my friendship with Winnie and my relationship with Lee might have been, but I think it would have been more of a scheduling issue than anything else. I concluded that competing with my metamour for time with a second shared lover was not attractive. My life was complex enough without adding another logistical and emotional layer.

Sometimes I wonder if the guy we both dated went on to have any more poly experiences. For the unmarried men I have dated for whom I was their first or one of their first polyamorous partners, after we went our separate ways, what taste did polyamory leave? I know at least a couple went on to pursue monogamous relationships. That led me to think I was a pit stop in their travels along the standard narrative speedway. Did they wish they could be polyamorous with their current girlfriends or wives? Did they feel constrained by monogamy? Did they cheat? Did they ever suggest open relationships to their partners? If so, what happened?

I like to think that for the most part, their experiences with me were positive and that our time together exposed them to a relationship that was joyful and fulfilling, at least for a while.

Or maybe they thought I was a freak and just hung around for the mind-blowing sex.

* * *

Winnie welcomed me sleeping over at her home with Lee, especially when it afforded her the ability to stay at her date's house or even go away for the weekend, which she did at least once, because we were home with their daughter. I had grown fond of Winnie and Lee's rambunctious munchkin. Will was a teen then, and I liked temporarily slipping back in time to those giggly, preschool, crayon- and Cheerio-filled days. It was a joy to read to her and hear her stumble over my name in her little kid way or shyly run from me—and, later, to me. She was the Easter egg of the relationship, unexpectedly pulling me closer in. Seeing Lee interact with his daughter made my affection for him grow. There was something alluring about a dad cooking pancakes and bacon and patiently letting his kid jockey for stirring privileges. Yes, she woke us up at ungodly hours, and Lee and I missed out on morning sex, but on balance, I forgave her.

One morning, as Lee, his daughter, and I were finishing breakfast, Winnie came home from her date and joined us at the table. I felt like a member of their freaky family, just a bit. It had not occurred to me how unwelcome I felt in Sylvia and Hank's home, even when I had permission to be there, until I lived the contrast. Lee was aware that I was dating Hank. He let me tell him as much or as little as I felt comfortable with, and that was not much.

One evening, I came over to Lee's house, and before I even sat down, he told me about his relationship and eventual breakup with his long-term girlfriend, whom he had been dating when he met Winnie. He also related a story of a female coworker who had a crush on him, whom he felt he had treated with less compassion than he wished he had. I figured that he was sharing these stories as his way of inviting me into his world, showing himself, being vulnerable. I knew that when he was done, I should do the same. If I failed to, then we would be on uneven footing. I imagined that he might have confided in Winnie, something akin to "I like Natalie, but she doesn't let me in, not all the way. I'm not sure what to do about it, other than be myself and provide as safe a place as I can for her to be herself." Lee's transparency cast a glare on my reticence.

I dated Hank and Lee at the same time for only three months, but the shadow Hank threw on my relationship with Lee was omnipresent. At a time when Lee was open and receptive to having me in his life, I was freshly wounded. By the time I was more healed from Hank's parting shots, Lee's life was changing.

Lee and I had dated for about eight months when he got a new job. His work became more demanding, he traveled a lot, and he was always on call. Not only did his work life change and his family move into a new home, but there were stresses in his marital relationship. He had less time for his family, his friends, and me. He seemed less happy. His carefree demeanor was overtaken by workaholism.

I tried to be understanding. I deferred to his job, family, and friends over me. I tended to withdraw when I sensed that someone did not have time for me. I bristled at feeling like an obligation. That was not sexy; that was pathetic.

A few months after Lee's job change, I was on my way to meet him for a rare evening out together in the city while Winnie was at home with their daughter. I had been looking forward to seeing Lee because we had not been alone together in weeks. He called me as I was driving, so I let the call go to voicemail. At a stop light, I played his message. I heard him sigh that a family situation had come up and he had to cancel our date. I could hear the frustration and apology in his voice. Still, I was irritated, all dressed up with no place to go. I made a U-turn toward home. Eric was on a date, so that made me feel even more abandoned.

Stuff happens. Grow up and stop being a brat, I chastised myself.

Eric and I had planned a cookout for the day following the canceled date with Lee, specifically during weekend daylight hours so that both Winnie and Lee could attend and bring their daughter. We had about a dozen adults in our backyard with a few kids in tow.

Not much was said about the night before. I decided I would not be anything less than understanding and forgiving, even though, as the afternoon progressed, I felt more and more like an afterthought, less and less like Lee's girlfriend of a year. I asked him if everyone was okay. They were. A car had hit their parked car. Lee was dealing with a work emergency and was in a sour mood. We exchanged no more than a dozen words during the cookout.

Some of the guests knew we were polyamorous, and some did not. Will still didn't. While our polyamory was not a state secret with the group of invited friends, I didn't broadcast it. I walked into the kitchen from the backyard to see Winnie talking to a friend of a friend of mine. Lee happened to walk in behind me. Winnie must have been explaining to the party guest how she knew me because I heard her say cheerfully, "Natalie is my husband Lee's girlfriend."

I felt the air being sucked from the room. I busied myself at the kitchen sink, my back to Winnie. The friend Winnie was talking to raised her eyebrows but said nothing I could hear over the rush of blood to my head and water to the sink. I almost said aloud in my best Inigo Montoya voice, *I don't think that means what you think it means,* because I was not feeling like Lee's girlfriend at that moment.

Hearing Winnie use that label made me wonder what I was to Lee and what we were to each other. He used to message me because he was thinking about me and wanted to see me, but lately, I felt that he was ticking off the box that asked: *Have you checked in with the girlfriend?* Yes, okay, next chore.

The following week, while Lee was on work travel, I texted him. "I miss the flirting."

"Thank you for saying how you're feeling," Lee responded. "Until you said you were noticing that I wasn't as engaged, I hadn't realized how what was happening at home was affecting you and affecting us."

Lee and I met at a coffee shop and discussed where things stood. He told me that Winnie was having personal difficulties that impacted him, their relationship, and their homelife. The upshot was that he had not been able to connect with me on anything other than a superficial level for months, but he had been so head down, so nose to the grindstone, that he had not realized how absent he was from our relationship.

I did not feel secondary or even tertiary. I felt less, like a ghost. I blamed myself somewhat. I had not gone out of my way to create a special space for us. I had struggled with how to define what Lee and I had. While Lee and Winnie regularly referred to me as his girlfriend, I had been reluctant to label it. I was not sure if that was fallout from being Hank's girlfriend—we had broken up months ago by then—or that I just didn't connect with Lee that way. Perhaps I didn't know what being a girlfriend looked like except for how it looked with Hank, and I knew it was not that, for better or for worse.

Being Hank's girlfriend had been a full-time job. It consumed my days, my head, and my emotional health. I liked Lee, and I enjoyed our time together physically and socially. He was sharp and compassionate, and I respected his opinions, even if I didn't always agree with them. He was a good guy, but I didn't let him into my psyche deep enough to find out if we could be more than friends and lovers.

As it turned out, guarding myself to some extent was apt foresight. When we finally met up to talk, Lee told me that he was unable to be to me what he wanted. The disconnect he was feeling at home with Winnie left him no heart space for anyone else. While Lee's words did not exactly parrot Hank's, they felt achingly close. I was saddened to learn that interpersonal matters were weighing on Lee. I supported him in turning his full attention to Winnie.

His words stung some, but not a lot. I was ready for his "it's not you, it's me" speech. I was always ready for it because that was just how it worked sometimes, especially with hierarchical polyamory.

Whatever the relationship label, sometimes those in it want to, or need to, focus on one partner more than another, and sometimes even to the exclusion of another. Lee and Winnie were married. They had a child together. I planted my feet firmly in the camp of "Certainly, I understand. Do what you need to do. Winnie takes priority, no question" because I could not avoid thinking that Eric might do the same to his girlfriend if he needed to devote more time to me.

What bothered me was that Lee's pulling away and the distance growing between us had started six months previously for reasons he did not share with me, even though they affected me. Thus, after expressing compassion about Winnie's problems, I told him that I did not like being left in the dark.

I was not angry or overly upset. That took energy I was not willing to part with. I was resigned. Polyamory appeared to bring with it a lot of breakups. Before I opened my marriage, I had not broken up with anyone in more than twenty years. Then it happened twice in nine months.

I let a few tears fall as Lee apologized. He was trying to be sweet. We did not prolong the farewell.

17.

The Mono-Poly Conundrum

More than one polyamory commentator, writer, and podcaster has said it: *Date your species.* When I first heard that directive, I had no idea what it meant, but it was said with such wearily voiced authority that I figured I'd better listen up.

Dating your species means polyamorous folks date polyamorous folks, and monogamous folks date monogamous folks, and if you cross those definitional lines, be prepared for Drama with a capital D.

That is not as simple as it sounds because the line between self-identifications is not always solid or even apparent. It can be like the painted lines dividing a highway. At some points, there is a double yellow. Do not cross! At some points, there is a break. Pass with care. Then there are the dotted or broken lines. Do your thing; just don't hurt anyone if you can help it.

I've dated guys who did not identify as polyamorous. They were fully aware from day one that I did. Even if they did not ask, I laid it all out. I figured if they knew that's how I rolled, and they chose to date me, they must be cool with polyamory, at least to some extent, right?

Wrong—or maybe sometimes right, and sometimes right for a bit, and then not, and occasionally awesomely right. Sometimes the guys were just confused.

I went out with Nico during the year I dated Lee. He had been in a long-term relationship that had ended within the past year, and he appeared to be interested in taking a break from serial monogamy. (Have we heard this tune before?) We met on a dating site.

"You read in my profile that I am married and polyamorous, right?"

"I did," he responded. "I think polyamory is very evolved and what I'm looking for."

Nico wooed me hard, taking me to offbeat bars and restaurants where the decibel level was low enough for us to talk and get to know each other. When we did connect physically, it was intense. I was not sure if it was good intense, as in "Let's do that again," or just "Fuck, that was intense, I need a breather to evaluate."

While in his bathroom regrouping, I noticed an abandoned clip-on nametag next to the sink. I recognized the printed acronym for an organization that Lee was affiliated with, or so I thought. I asked Nico if it was that group. It was.

"I think I may know someone in that group," I said.

"Yeah? Ooh, let me guess!"

Really? I thought. *We are playing that game?*

Apparently, that professional community was a small one. As I was learning more every day, so was polyamory.

He guessed correctly on his first try, probably because he knew Lee well enough to have invited him to his wedding to a woman he broke up with right before the nuptials. Lee was more public than me about his open marriage, and I guessed he was one of the few local polyamorous people Nico knew. That I was dating Lee seemed to delight Nico. The sudden gleam in his eye nearly blinded me. I felt a bit like a prize pig at the state fair.

The next time I saw Lee, I told him I had been out with Nico a few times. Lee seemed cool with it, although I did detect a raised eyebrow. Lee and Nico could not have been more physically different—Lee was tall, thin, and angular with blue eyes and light brown hair; Nico was average height, heavier build, dark-eyed, dark-haired, and covered with a pelt of fur that surprised me once we undressed—and there were other differences.

I sensed that Lee did not approve of how Nico had treated his former fiancée with the last-minute breakup, but, being a gentleman, he did not go into details. I felt a little judged even though Lee said, "Nico is a good guy. I wish you two well."

I wanted to add, "I am not sure I am going to see him again, but I wanted to let you know I saw him since you two know each other, and I didn't want you to be blindsided because Nico seemed like the kind a guy who might elbow you and say, 'Hey, dude, guess who I'm seeing?'"

I debated about whether to keep seeing Nico and concluded that he would be a fun date buddy since he was single and more available. Lee had more trouble extracting himself from his family and work obligations to get together as often as I would have liked.

Nico suggested that we meet for lunch, and I accepted. He canceled at the last minute, saying that a conflict had arisen. No big deal. We had some back-and-forth messaging and then a lot of silence. It felt odd that he did not contact me to reschedule since he had been so into me and had been the one to propose the lunch date, but I understood. People get busy. I was also busy with Eric, with Lee, with life.

A couple of weeks later, I was at a formal military dinner with Eric, and I checked my phone while in the restroom. Nico had texted.

"I'd like to talk. Can I call you?"

"Can't now," I responded.

Hearing nothing the next day, I followed up. "What's up? You can tell me by text." When a millennial asks if they can "talk" versus "text," you know something is up, and I figured I knew what it was.

"Hey, so I wanted you to know that, yes, I canceled lunch because work is a nightmare, but also because I started seeing someone. I want to see where it goes as a monogamous relationship, so I can't keep seeing you even though I think you're great."

Gritting my teeth and rolling my eyes, I inhaled and texted, "Understood. Good luck!"

"Thanks!" he replied. End of story.

I noticed he took his profile off the dating site because our chat history had a notation that "this profile is no longer active." Some weeks later, his profile was back up. *That relationship didn't last long.*

Because I wasn't that attached to Nico, I didn't think his goodbye text would affect me much, but after I had thought about it more, I felt like the good-time girl you date before you find the girl to build your white picket fence around.

Nico's final texts put me on notice for the next time I was tempted to date someone else new to polyamory. I vowed to figure out what I wanted from the dating relationship and to communicate that upfront. My next relationship was a step in that direction.

CJ entered my life after Hank and after Lee—after a lot had happened in my poly evolution. When we met, I was upfront about what I was doing, what I wanted, and who I was. I hit him with Polyamory 101 immediately. He met Eric when he picked me up at the house for our second date. The doorbell rang while I was finishing getting ready upstairs. Before I could hurry down the stairs, I heard Eric open the door to greet CJ. Then I heard Eric say, "So you're the guy who's here to fuck my wife."

I froze on the stairs. I couldn't see Eric's face, but I knew he was yanking CJ's chain. Did CJ? As I was about to bound down and intervene, CJ's laughter rose to meet me. I heard Eric's laughter, and I saw them exchange handshakes. On our date, CJ told me about his and his ex-wife's disillusionment with each other and the dissolution of their marriage. CJ was the first man I had heard talk openly about therapy and how it had helped him. He told me he was going through a period of exploration after his marriage, trying to figure out what he wanted next. That made sense to me.

For my part, I told CJ that while I liked sex, that was not enough.

"I am looking for a dating relationship where we go out together and are part of each other's lives. I don't like being a dirty secret. If you aren't in a place for that, I understand, but I want to know that now before we get attached."

He nodded, his dimples deepening and his blue eyes sparkling with affirmation. "Yes, I love relationships," he said. I had never heard any guy say they loved relationships. "That's what I want, too," he continued. "I've dated a poly woman before. I am on board with each of us not being jealous of the relationships we have with others. I like you and find you attractive. We are on the same page."

We talked about polyamory a lot on those first few dates. I was trying to probe his poly-compatibility level. I was ready for a longer-term relationship. I missed the strong physical and emotional connection, fun outings, and daily communication I had enjoyed with Hank. I missed trading sexts, snarky jabs, and songs we liked.

CJ was a scientist in his mid-thirties, had no kids, was attractive in a short-haired, clean-cut way, fit, seemingly self-aware, and a good communicator. He was recently divorced from his college sweetheart because she fell out of love with him. Ouch. He was close to his churchgoing family. CJ and his brothers were best friends. He was trying to figure out what came next, which was probably kids and a wife, but not right away.

He was interested in what polyamory meant and how it might suit him. He was jazzed at the prospect of something so different than his years of vanilla monogamy. To him, I seemed full of potential adventures. We started frenzied texting, sexting, and thirst-trap selfie swapping despite his crazy work schedule. He employed more emoticons than I knew existed. I was exhilarated to be *that* woman—the one who excites and titillates, the one whom dreams are made of.

We attended a theater performance that bordered on experimental, which was a kind way to say that either we were too bourgeois to appreciate the existential themes, or the play sucked. After the show, we drank beer at a crowded rooftop bar and talked about polyamory, his divorce, my marriage, sexploits, relationships, favorite foods, and our bucket list of travel destinations. We made plans to see another show (hopefully better!), and I bought tickets. We kept texting and trading stories and fantasies. I was feeling the high of new relationship energy that I had been missing.

On the day of the play, he texted me, saying, "I can't do it."

I responded, "Can't do what—can't make the show? Is work intruding?"

"Not exactly," he said. "Well, yes, work is insane, and I haven't slept much, but it's more that I am having trouble with the idea of polyamory. I can't quite get my head around it. I thought I could do it, but right now, I need self-care."

My first inclination was to tell him how inconsiderate it was to cancel at noon, leaving me holding tickets, because he was doing a one-eighty about relationship dynamics on three hours of sleep, and, oh yeah, to tell him to fuck the hell off.

Instead, I took a breath. I talked to Eric. I told him what CJ had said, and I asked for his opinion. I asked Eric because I knew myself. I knew that my instinctive reaction was to get my back up. I didn't want to do that. I wanted to be better at dating—kinder and more patient.

Eric said, "Tell him that he should keep the date, and you guys can have a pleasant evening. You can talk about your relationship the next time you see each other."

"What? I should beg him to go out with me when he just said he was feeling conflicted and had the nerve to cancel at the last minute? That seems pathetic."

Eric sighed. "Natalie, it is not pathetic. Do you want to see him?"

"Yes, but I am not going to beg—no damn way. I am not hard up, and I deserve better treatment."

"I don't see that as begging. I see it as keeping the date, which is what you want, right?"

"I guess."

"I don't mind giving you my opinion, but if you don't want it, don't ask me for it."

"I do want your opinion," I said. "You're right. I want to see him. I like him. That's why this hurts. And I feel stupid, which is my least favorite emotion."

CJ and I went to the show and then back to his place. I saw his house and met his dog, both of which he got in the divorce. He told me about his foray into winemaking and presented me with a bottle of red. I was touched. The label bore a likeness of his chocolate Labrador.

I didn't know what, if anything, would come of us, but I was drawn to his honesty and his impish smile. When we kissed in his living room, and I felt it in my toes, I took his hand and led him to the bedroom. Even if that one night of intimacy was all we would have, I could not claim to be blindsided. He had told me who he was and what he was struggling with. I left his house with a wistful smile, feeling flushed and cared for. Polyamory might not be his path, but I was still happy ours had crossed. Over the years, we remained friends—and occasionally lovers. A few months later, at a kink conference, I introduced him to erotic rope bondage and to the woman who would become his wife.

18.
Downshifting and Exhaling

At the end of the summer, my one-year relationship with Lee ended, which was a few years into my dating separately from Eric, and I started seeing a thirtysomething economist. We had fun eating oysters, attending plays, and almost breaking his bed. To date, he holds the blue ribbon for the least expected follow-up sentence to "There's something I should tell you before we go any further," said while we were still vertical in the dark of his bedroom.

"I don't have testicles. I had cancer, and they were removed." He said this as a simple fact. Clearly, he had said it before.

"Are you okay with that?" he continued while I faced him in my underwear, my dress already on the floor.

I paused for a beat, digesting the information.

"Sure." I shrugged. *They just get in the way*, I thought. We tumbled onto his bed.

He liked us to hang out while he and his housemates smoked pot and watched one of the post-Kirk and Spock *Star Trek* series. It was not my idea of fun, although I could see the allure of watching aliens while getting baked.

In my forties, I was woefully naïve about drugs. I had fantasies of someday trying psychedelics and hearing toads who glistened like oil slicks speak to me before melting into rainbow-streaked puddles. I had no idea if that was what happened on mushrooms or acid. I probably saw it in a movie. Hank was going to be my drug partner since he had tried them all and knew enough to keep me safe, or so he had told me.

This single guy was polyamorous and dating multiple women. "I'm in that sweet spot in my mid-thirties where I can date older and younger women," he told me. "I have to say I am enjoying it."

"I can see that," I said. "I can date older and younger as well, although younger seems to work out better for me."

But from the wistful way he talked about his ex-girlfriend, who might have been moving to DC, he seemed nostalgic for his former monogamous relationship. That made me think that for some people, polyamory functioned more as a placeholder until they found their "one and only." To me, that was not polyamory. That was dating around until you found the monogamous relationship that worked for you.

I surmised that slapping the polyamory label on what my mother's generation called "playing the field" made a guy feel less like a player. But if you were not fully engaging in the relationship aspects of dating—caring, affection, time, and commitment—and it was more about hooking up and bonking until you found a monogamous relationship, that did not seem like polyamory to me.

A few months later, when the *Sayonara, sweetheart* came, his recitation of "I am not in the headspace for this" sounded to me like single-dude code for *This is starting to feel like a relationship with responsibilities, and that is not what I signed up for. I just wanted some fun and figured you being married would free me from any emotional labor.* That his brush-off was delivered by text made me feel officially initiated into the new millennium of romance, such that it was. We broke up via a green speech bubble on my phone. At least it was benign. No Hank-like vitriol, so that was an improvement.

After the summer ended, along with my relationships with Hank, Lee, and the guy with no balls, I dated a bit, but nothing amounted to much of a relationship. I made an unexpected connection with the chef de cuisine at a white tablecloth restaurant, thus granting me entry into an unfamiliar world—the workaholic, obsessive, and too often abusive nature of fine-dining kitchen work. In part because of his evening schedule, we saw each other infrequently, and our relationship petered out. We had little to talk about other than his work. We remained friends, and I visited his restaurant occasionally. He would bring me a new menu item and ask my opinion. If he was not overwhelmed in the kitchen, we could talk at the bar before the dinner crowd came in.

While we were dating, Eric adored the chef's culinary skills. I had never seen him swoon so much over food. The chef enjoyed feeding us as we savored the decadence of his creations. Even our son Will was a fan. As a teenager, Will was typically uninterested in accompanying his parents out to eat, but it was a different story when we said we were going to the chef's place. Then he was all in.

During times when Will was not with us, and the chef visited our table to see how we were enjoying the dishes, sometimes with Marianne at our table, Eric delighted in saying into the chef's ear, with a conspiratorial grin, "Bro, if you keep feeding us this fabulous food, you can bang my wife as much as you want." I would blush and hush him. Then we would all laugh.

Eric embraced most of my partners as instantly beloved metamours, whether they fed us or not. In this way, Eric made polyamory easier for me. He rarely experienced the jealousy or prickliness that I did toward metamours. It was only when he felt that my partners were treating me poorly or were a threat to our relationship that his warm welcomes chilled, like the evenings I waited for Felix—Mr. Failure to Appear who I'd met on the CollarMe site—to be free or when Hank's breakup words made me cry.

About six months after Lee and I parted, and four months after Eric and Marianne split, I met Trevor. I had reactivated my dating app, and Trevor's goofy pictures and upbeat attitude piqued my interest. Our first date was over a shared love of messy Texas barbecue. He offered to pay, but I had ordered a pound to go for my boys at home—Eric and Will—so that didn't seem right. He insisted on walking me to the train station, which was out of his way. The awkward pause before we parted was thankfully short, and the goodbye kiss was promising. He texted me almost immediately about wanting to get together again.

In his late twenties, Trevor was younger than me by about twenty years. My attempts at dating guys my age had led nowhere. I accepted what worked for me. Trevor and I were comfortable with each other. We talked easily about our families, living in Texas where hunting and barbeque were a way of life, and our preference for liberal politics. We connected physically, spending hours exploring each other's bodies in all the rooms of his apartment. When we were together,

I felt affection and desire flowing easily in both directions. Trevor had briefly dated a polyamorous woman before me and told me that he did not get jealous of her other partners.

Before driving to his place in the city, I would choose racy underwear and a dress that hugged me in a way that made me feel pretty. I would strap on high-heeled sandals since he was a head taller than me. On the drive over, I would picture how he would greet me, his hands on me immediately. My right foot would become heavier on the accelerator.

On one visit, I had barely crossed his apartment threshold when he kissed me and hoisted me onto the sofa arm. He kneeled as if to propose.

"Trevor, what are you doing?" I laughed.

"I want to properly welcome you to my humble abode."

He pushed up my dress. I was flushed with his intense attention and decadent oral skills. The dizziness I felt may have also been due to my head being thrown back as I propped myself up on my elbows. Whatever the cause, I was not arguing with the effect.

"Mm," he said with a grin, standing up. "Appetizer is over. Shall we cook?"

Trevor subscribed to a service that delivered all the raw ingredients and step-by-step instructions for a meal for two. He was the first guy with whom I had cooked a complete dinner. In my household, I made most meals. Eric grilled. I was intrigued by the prospect of preparing a meal side-by-side with my date, like all those rom-coms where the guy invites the girl over to his place and impresses her with his farmer's market produce, culinary skills, and wine choice, thereby winning her over and, usually, bedding her.

Trevor pulled the individual heat-sealed packets of chicken, vegetables, and spices from his otherwise barren, single-guy fridge. He propped the instruction page on the counter and retrieved the appropriately sized pots and pans. He pulled out a cutting board and a serious-looking chef's knife.

"What can I do to help?" I asked. I watched over his shoulder as he read the recipe card.

"There's not that much to do. I was going to chop the onion and garlic."

"I can preheat the oven and get the potatoes ready," I offered.

"Sounds good." He smiled.

Trevor gave his full attention to the cutting board. He uniformly diced the onions and crushed and chopped the garlic cloves.

Huh, I thought, *he's got more impressive knife skills than I would have thought.*

Done with my minor chore, I perched myself on the kitchen counter next to him. Watching him concentrate on making the vegetables yield to his large blade was sexy.

"I'm setting the timer for eight minutes for the chicken to cook in the oven before finishing it off in the pan."

"Eight minutes. Roger that, chef." I saluted two fingers to my brow.

He kissed me. "Think I can make you come before the buzzer?"

I laughed. "I don't know. You already did. I'm still wet, but I would never turn down your talented tongue."

"Challenge accepted," he said. "Scoot forward a bit."

My underwear was still off from the last round. I moved my hips to the edge of the counter and leaned back. I could get used to this, but with one eye on the oven timer, I had a hard time fully concentrating. I closed my eyes and tried to let myself melt into his mouth.

Bzzz! went the timer.

"Oh, I was so close," I breathed.

Trevor rose and kissed my mouth. "Ah, well, still fun." He pulled the pan out of the oven.

"Definitely," I agreed. "Cooking shows could increase viewership tenfold if they followed your lead. We could call it *Cunnilingus in the Kitchen*."

"Or *Blowing Your Way to Mind-blowing Breakfasts*," he said.

I hopped down from the counter, and we finished cooking the meal. After eating dinner cross-legged in front of his living room coffee table, we made our way to his tiny bedroom and had dessert.

When we started dating, I told Trevor that I had once asked a guy I was on a first date with, after we had sex in his apartment, whether it was safe to walk alone for several blocks at midnight to where my car was parked on a city side street. I assumed he would offer to walk with me. He had said, "Oh, you'll be fine," before closing his front door. I had walked quickly to my parked car, my heart racing and my keys in hand. As I was unlocking my car door, the guy texted, "Did you get to your car okay?" I thought, *If I hadn't, I would be lying on the street bleeding out and unable to answer this text, so what is the point exactly?* I chose not to see him again.

Trevor unfailingly, and unsolicited, walked me to my car each time I came over. Often, I parked almost within sight of his front door, and I told him it was not necessary for him to get dressed to walk me across the street. He would just shrug. "It's no problem. Of course, I'll walk you. Gives me more time to spend with you, anyway." That meant I got an extra goodbye kiss at my car that sent me home to Eric in a flush of goodwill, as well as postcoital euphoria.

I could not help but think, *Someone raised him right. Southern boy with good manners.* Later, another partner would tell me that it was not fair to hold it against someone if I didn't ask for what I wanted. If I wanted the guy to walk me to my car because it made me feel safer, then I should open my mouth and ask. Point taken, I resolved to do so.

I liked the time I spent with Trevor, but between his full-time job, his reserve military duties, and whatever introvert space he needed, we did not have as much time together as I would have liked. We talked of getting together for outside-the-apartment activities like a movie or a hike, but he ended up not having time for them. He did not include me in get-togethers with his friends. He did not introduce me to his best friend, who lived next door to him.

At the time I was dating him, it was a rarity that my lovers and my husband not only met but also spoke to each other at length and in-depth, so I remember clearly the dinner when Eric and Trevor met. They worked in similar career fields and were both in the military reserve, so they had a lot in common. Eric, while more advanced in his field, related effortlessly to Trevor. For his part, Trevor impressed me with his comfort and maturity. They geeked out about their work and military service. I felt a little excluded, but I was shyly smiling the whole time, just listening. I was happy.

After we finished dinner, Eric offered Trevor a ride home. We three were walking to the car when Eric said, more to Trevor than to me, "You know, I'm cool with PDA, so feel free." Emboldened, I took Trevor's hand, and we held on like teenagers until we reached the car. We drove to Trevor's place, and I walked him to his door while Eric waited behind the wheel. "No rush," he said.

On his doorstep, Trevor and I kissed. I felt my chest swell, both from Trevor's kiss and from feeling bathed in Eric's compersion. I knew as I said goodbye to Trevor that Eric was waiting patiently in the car, without possessiveness, without jealousy; with love.

As we drove home, Eric remarked on Trevor's smarts and good looks. "I am happy for you, Natalie."

"I doubt it will last," I sighed. "Trevor doesn't have much time for me."

Eric patted my thigh in that "my wife is hot" way he had been doing for years. "From what I could see, the guy is pretty smitten with you, for good reason."

I put my hand on his and let his love wash over me.

That dinner was the last time I saw Trevor before he left for an overseas military assignment. We were separated by thousands of miles and a tangible lack of touch, but thinking about him made me smile. We kept in touch by text, email, and sexy chats. I sent him care packages with homemade cookies and a thumb drive holding not-safe-for-work photos and videos. I looked forward to his return and finding out whether we could pick up where we left off. I didn't know if we could, but even if we never did, I thought I would be at peace with it. I was glad polyamory had brought Trevor into my life.

19.

Coming Clean

Will was in high school when I got a call from Eric. I was on a work trip and in line to check into my hotel.

"This funny thing happened. Leah and I were in the basement while Will was out, and—this is the funny part—he must have come home without us realizing it because I got a text: 'Hey, Dad, it sounds like someone is having loud sex in the basement.'"

I waited for the funny part.

Will had been searching for a resupply of Double Stuf Oreos, which I kept on a shelf in the basement with overflow pantry items. Eric had locked the door to the basement, but Will had opened it with the interior key pin we still kept perched on a door ledge from when he was young and accidentally—or on purpose—locked himself inside a room. Halfway down the stairs, he heard Leah. Will did not turn the corner to the area where the sounds came from, thankfully, but went back upstairs and texted his dad.

Eric responded to Will's text. "That would be me. Be right up."

I could hear the smirk in Eric's voice when he asked me what I wanted to do. "Come on, Natalie, this could have just as easily happened to you."

"No," I said from the hotel lobby. "I always remember to restock the upstairs snacks when *I* have company. Let's talk to Will together when I get home tomorrow night."

About ten minutes later, Eric texted me: "Talked to Will. All good."

I called Eric.

Eric told me that Leah was mortified, but he convinced her to come upstairs for a brief appearance before dashing out.

"I didn't want to wait because I didn't want him to think I was cheating on you and that the stability of his home and family was at risk," Eric said. "I told him that we had an agreement where we both could date and have sex with other people."

According to Eric, Will shrugged, said "It's none of my business," and went up to his room. Eric was satisfied. In fact, he seemed a little smug: *See, Natalie, you were worried for nothing.*

All those years of guilt and fretting over whether and when to tell Will, what to say, and how it would affect him crumbled into a heap, like so much impotent ash after a roaring fire.

I realized that I was relieved. I was also impressed that Will had been so unconcerned, as if, perhaps, we had modeled behavior and attitudes over the years that led him to a level of comfort and acceptance with the news. Or, more likely, his parents' dating life did not affect him, so he did not spend time examining it.

After I came home from my trip, I waited a few days to let Will digest the information. I knocked on his door.

"Yeah," he said. I came in and sat on his bed.

"That thing that happened while I was away, do you have any questions, anything you want to talk about?" I asked. "Or would you rather not talk about it at all?"

Will was quiet, thinking. "No," he said, "not at the moment."

I offered poly books and websites if he wanted to know more. He shrugged, disinterested.

"Do you have homework?" I asked.

"Some," he said. "I'm working on it."

I was halfway out the door when he stopped me in *Columbo* just-one-more-thing style.

"Mom?"

"Yes," I said, turning back from the doorway.

"Do you have sex with Hank?"

I hesitated a second. "Yes," I said.

Will was quiet.

"Does that bother you?" I asked.

"No," he said. "That makes sense."

Internally, I winced. Finally, he could reconcile why Hank and I hung out, seeing as how "you are not nerdy at all, Mom," and Hank was.

The following year, Will was home from college on spring break, eating my homemade chicken and sausage gumbo, heaping on the rice. Sitting on the kitchen counter in a giant box was a chocolate Easter bunny I had bought for him, even though he had long outgrown the springtime baskets. I knew he loved the bunnies, eating the ears first with a carnivorous chomp.

"Mom, I had a hard time believing in the Spring Bunny for years after you were still pretending there was one," said Will, "but I didn't say anything because I thought if the Spring Bunny isn't real, then Mom is lying to me, and Mom wouldn't lie to me. When I found out that you were lying to me, my worldview shifted."

"My pretending there is a Spring Bunny who brings you candy and toys—*that* was the watershed lie of your life?" I shook my head. "And here I was worried that finding out that your father and I had an open marriage would have been that."

That opened the door to discussion. I was curious about what was rattling around in his head about polyamory. He listened as I prattled on about how nice it was to be able to enjoy doing things with others that his dad did not like to do, and vice versa. I had recently taken a trip with Wesley, whom Will had met (and who will reappear in chapter 21 of this book), to India, a subcontinent Eric had no desire to visit. I used that as an example, as well as how Leah and Eric went camping more often than I was interested in going.

My son smiled and nodded. "I can't see being with only one person my whole life. An open marriage makes sense."

"I'm relieved," I said. "It's important to know you have choices in how you live your life. I struggled with when to tell you about Dad and me and decided to tell you if you asked. I figured that would let me know you were ready to hear it."

He said, "Mom, that assumes that I would have been comfortable asking you even if I suspected something. I might have kept it to myself and assumed wrongly that either you or Dad were being dishonest with each other."

"Valid point," I said. "I think that discovering polyamory was a relief for your dad."

"Because he was attracted to other women?" Will asked. "I get that. It's natural to be attracted to others."

"Your father has always been a flirt," I said, laughing. "He's always liked women."

"Yeah. It is good to know Dad and you have an agreement."

With that as a segue, I asked, "Did you ever think that Dad was dating Marianne?"

"Yes," he said, "but I never would have guessed about you and Hank."

I laughed and said, "Because we are so different, and he is so much cooler than I am?"

Will smiled.

"Hank and I aren't dating anymore," I said. "He has a new girlfriend."

"Aw," he said, in a way that told me he was a sweet kid who loved his mom.

"Thanks, bug. It's fine. As you said, Hank and I have always been very different, and once his wife moved out, he was reexamining his life."

Will said, "I hadn't realized how different I was from Hank until we talked about political philosophy that time."

"Yes, I remember when you hijacked my date to talk about communism," I said.

I had assumed Will and Hank stuck to nerding about video games and comics. I let their online contact be between them. When Hank told me he thought "the boy should be told" about us, he respected my decision even though he disagreed.

I like to think that Will experienced the positive nature of our lifestyle before he knew about it by living in a house that welcomed a kaleidoscope of people. After the reveal, I worried that he might have wondered whether anyone we introduced him to from then on was a romantic interest. I don't think it mattered to him because he never asked when Eric or I kissed a partner hello or cuddled on the sofa while watching a movie.

We were still the parents who nagged him about school and chores. We were still the same old parents he had seen kissing each other in the kitchen and canoodling on the couch all his life. We still spent time as a couple, the couple we had been since we fell in love when Cyndi Lauper and shoulder pads were in vogue. Will could still depend on us to love and support him, whether we were monogamous or not.

20.
The Future of Polyamory

The thread that pulled me to Bennett was his writerly aspiration. He had developed a fantasy trilogy he likened to *Game of Thrones*. He was editing the first book and had a detailed outline for the next two. He was also writing a postwar dystopic feminist novel about a world where women controlled the government while roving bands of men wreaked havoc. He would read his work to me, and I would read mine to him. I thought he wrote well, especially for someone only a few years out of college.

When we met, Bennett told me his dead-end retail job was just until he published his book, which he sounded casually certain would make him scads of money. I admired his confidence in the quality and marketability of his writing. I struggled with both.

His girlfriend Lana was in her senior year of college. Bennett had an old-soul view of himself, which I found endearing and eye-rollingly naïve. Even though he was only a few years older than Lana, he told me he felt so more adult because he was out in the world. I pictured him reclining in a Hefner-esque smoking jacket and puffing on a pipe. Their plan, he told me, was to move to wherever she went for graduate school because he could write anywhere. In the meantime, Lana lived in an apartment a few miles from Bennett. Lana was supported by her parents, who had threatened to withdraw funding if she and Bennett moved in together.

I usually met Bennett at the two-bedroom apartment he shared with two guys. Bennett used the dining room as his bedroom. In the narrow doorway that led from the kitchen to the dining room, he had hung a blue and white striped bed sheet. Lacking a fourth wall, the other side of his crash space was separated from the living room by a rattan tri-fold panel you might find at World Market that stood three feet shy of the ceiling. His bed, desk, office chair, and dresser filled his small space. The window ledge served as a counter for beer bottles, water glasses, and condom packets. A self-made map of the fantasy world in his book series stretched across the entirety of one of the three walls of his room. He used the map as a reference to explain to me the intricate geopolitical machinations of his story.

On several occasions, I drove Bennett to Lana's apartment on my way home from our date. Lana would make dinner for them both if he and I had not already eaten. Lana and I saw each other only once. She, Bennett, Eric, and I had met for dinner at the beginning of my relationship with Bennett. Lana was a brown-eyed beauty with a lush mocha complexion. I was mesmerized by her looks and by her composure at meeting us. Bennett and Lana had been dating for a year or two. Ostensibly, both were open to dating others, but in practice, only Bennett dated on his own. They sometimes dated the same person simultaneously as a threesome.

According to Bennett, Lana was stressed by college and her looming future and didn't feel she had the bandwidth to date anyone except him. She resented his dating. This was partly because he had more time for it than she did. To hear Bennett tell it, everything would be better once she graduated because she would have the headspace and time to date. I was more doubtful, but hey, not my rodeo. More than once, I offered to meet Lana for coffee or a drink, just to be friendly. She politely put me off, saying she was too busy, but maybe sometime soon.

Bennett had been polyamorous since he was fifteen and first started having sex. He told me that polyamory was a natural state for him. He had tried monogamy after the pushback he got from friends and family for not following the standard narrative, but it had never worked for him. He was irritated by Lana's rules and control, which smacked of monogamy. They had argued about whether he had violated her rule of not dating someone from work when he had dated a customer from the shop where he and Lana worked. He continued to see the customer, but he didn't tell Lana, against my advice.

"How does she feel about you and me dating? Do you tell her?" I asked.

"Oh, she's cool with you," he said, smiling. "She likes you."

"Because I'm not a threat to your relationship?" *Like a young hottie you see behind her back*, I thought, even though I knew nothing about the customer.

He thought about it. "Maybe something like that. You are experienced at poly and are considerate to her. She appreciates that."

"I tried reaching out to her to get coffee or something," I continued, "but so far, it hasn't happened. I think it demystifies polyamory and calms anxieties if metamours have some kind of relationship. I don't want to push her, but I was not sure what vibe I was getting."

"I wouldn't worry about it," he said. "She's stressed about school and stuff."

Bennett was the youngest person I had met who identified unquestionably as polyamorous. While he craved connection, he did not want to limit those connections to one person, one gender, or one relationship. He told me that he did not see that as morally wrong, even though his perspective flew in the face of everything he had been taught. His first girlfriend in high school took it personally that he dated other girls and thought his being non-exclusive meant that she was somehow deficient. Her friends viewed him as an emotionally abusive jerk. Bennett's friends dismissed him as the guy who couldn't keep it in his pants. His family told him he was being irresponsible and selfish and that he should "pick one girl."

Bennett was an attractive, emotionally intelligent young white man who self-identified as a feminist and bisexual. He would also tell you without shame—and I wonder if he even realized how objectifying he sounded—that he only dated those who were different than him. Lana, for example, was biracial. I apparently qualified because I was much older than him.

I admit to being flattered by his attraction to me as a "sexy older woman" and dismissed it as a sidenote to us developing a relationship based on mutual interests and desires, but after a few months, I wondered if I was more a notch in his collection of trophied others and less a self-actualized person. That may be an overstatement and unfair to Bennett, because we did have great conversations about everything from sociology and politics to relationships and writing. But as time passed, we saw each other less and less, then not at all. Lana was graduating with her bachelor's degree. I was not privy to whether their plan to relocate for her graduate studies was afoot. It also became more difficult to plan time together. He had weekend retail shifts, and I worked a nine-to-five job.

While we dated, I was fascinated by Bennett's comfort in his poly skin. To me, he was the face of the twentysomethings who were embracing polyamory as a viable alternative to monogamy. Bennett liked sex, but he also sought intimacy and affection. He said he was in love with Lana, and I had no reason to doubt that. He spoke fondly of her and treated her with consideration as far as I could see—other than lying about his dating, which I was finding to be a recurring problem with men.

For real, what is with the lies men tell themselves to protect the feelings of their women? Eric used to do it with me. When he cheated on me with Katrina and Lorraine, he told me he wanted to be honest but did not want to hurt me. Hank did it with Sylvia and with me when he omitted full truths of how he was spending his time with each of us or whether Sylvia was displeased with me or him or us—"I am just trying to keep everyone happy"—and with the women he dated before us. I would like to have a word with whoever told men that women would rather be lied to "for their own good" than be told the truth.

When we parted, Bennett, the polyamorist, was still maturing—the human frontal cortex does not fully develop until the mid to late twenties. He was still learning the importance of honest and open communication, the value of which I reiterated to him often. I hoped that one day I would find that he had published his books in progress, and I would buy them all.

21.
Community

In 2016, I attended my first polyamory conference. It was conveniently located within driving distance of home. My intention was to meet polyamorous folks, hear from noted speakers, participate in seminars, and become more integrated into the polyamory community. Eric, to my delight, agreed to come with me.

I had local poly friends and acquaintances, and I had attended local polyamory talks and meetups, but I had not found a poly group that suited me. The weekly meetups were either small and awkward or too far away from where I lived.

One gathering met in the back room of a fast-casual salad shop under harsh fluorescent lighting. Eric and I sat on stiff plastic chairs while a genial gray-haired woman in braids led the group. She offered no specific discussion topic. Rather, we all introduced ourselves from where we sat at four-tops or two-tops, alone or with partners, and offered general thoughts. I sensed that the single guys were hoping to meet potential partners.

Another weeknight meetup was a forty-minute drive from our house. At least thirty people crowded into the host's living room to listen to a speaker. Eric and I made small talk with other polyamorous people, but we felt little connection. The ramblings that passed as questions were disjointed and unfocused. I was reminded of classmates who raised their hands to express a long-winded opinion rather than ask a question that would advance the discussion. We crossed that meetup off our list.

I was excited that the conference would afford me some distance from home and the opportunity to participate in a nationwide event. Maybe interacting with a broader cross-section of the polyamorous would yield a better understanding of how others practiced polyamory and an opportunity to relate to my people.

We arrived at the conference hotel on a Friday afternoon. Eric and I stood in a circle with the other attendees and played icebreaker games. We browsed vendor tables with books and CDs about polyamory, relationships, and sex. We scanned the schedule for the two days of seminars, activities, and evening events and highlighted some of interest. Topics included an Introduction to Polyamory, Communication Skills, a writing workshop, Polyamory and the Law, Tantric Poly, Dealing with Abuse, and Diversity in the Polyamory Community.

The conference also gave participants the chance to host impromptu sessions. The keynote speaker, a sex and relationship expert, was engaging, and I felt energized and ready to open myself up to the experiences of the weekend. After dinner in the hotel restaurant, Eric and I got ready for the evening's masquerade party.

In keeping with the theme, we dressed in club clothes and Mardi Gras masks. In the ballroom, a deejay played upbeat tunes. People, most of them paired up, were doing what you do at parties where you don't know anyone—chatting, people-watching, sipping drinks, maybe dancing. Some people played a mixer game, meeting people to fill squares on a card for "has traveled to South America" or "has been poly for less than a year."

For the mixer, I had un-Velcro'd myself from my default position at Eric's side. I wanted to get out there, be my polyamorous self, meet new people, and engage! The trip was my idea, after all. While Eric was comfortable striking up a conversation with anyone, I felt more drained making small talk, so after a few rounds of meet-new-people bingo, I migrated to the edge of the dance floor.

I listened to the music and nursed a drink, trying to appear approachable and vowing not to tether myself to Eric. *Smile, Natalie,* I thought. Standing almost at my elbow was a very tall, lanky guy. Through his bandit-style mask, I could see his blue-gray eyes and a generous smile.

"My partner isn't here yet," he said, "so I don't have anyone to dance with."

"This *is* a poly con," I pointed out, smiling at him. "You can ask someone else to dance." For me, that was extreme flirting.

He smiled in that way you do when you did not hear what the other person said but don't want to be rude by saying so, or when you did hear but don't want to be rude by saying you're not interested. Then he turned away.

After a minute or two, a song came on that I liked, so I stepped onto the parquet floor and started dancing. In the gothic, industrial, electronic music club scene I was familiar with, dancing alone to music that moved you was as natural as breathing. Eric and I did it all the time at home.

When I looked up, I saw the masked stranger grinning at me.

"May I dance with you?" he asked.

"Sure." I shrugged and smiled. When the song ended, we peeled off to escape the deejay's next pick, a slow tune that cleared the floor. Eric was standing nearby, beaming at me.

"Natalie," he said as he kissed my cheek, "I see you've met Wesley." My dance partner lifted his simple black fabric mask and introduced himself with a grin. "We met during the mixer," Eric said.

Wesley and I talked for a bit and then lost track of each other. I met a few more folks, including a poly blogger whose work I had admired for years. Eric and I did not stay at the masquerade too late. We had a full schedule the following day, and I was eager to be up early at our first poly conference.

At the first morning session, I spotted Wesley a row behind me. We nodded our recognition. The instructor told us to pair up for the workshop exercise. Eric and I tacitly agreed to find different partners so we could learn from new people. The presentation was on self-interest in relationships and used a game theory exercise called the Prisoner's Dilemma to show why two completely rational individuals might not cooperate, even when it appeared that it was in their best interests to do so.* The presenter posited that intelligent, self-interested people are motivated toward investing in healthy relationships and that short-term selfishness hurts an individual in the long run by losing the trust of valuable people.

I partnered with the guy sitting next to me for the first round and with a woman sitting a few seats over for the second round. For the third round, I saw Wesley over my shoulder, and he smiled and glanced down at the empty seat

* https://en.wikipedia.org/wiki/Prisoner's_dilemma explains the game theory in detail.

beside him. After we finished our round, Wesley said that he had played the game before. He expanded on the theory behind the game without arrogance or as if he were trying to impress me, although in retrospect, maybe he was trying just a little. Our hands touched briefly when we looked at what we had each written on our papers as part of the exercise. I felt a pleasant hum of electricity between us.

When the session ended, Eric found me and greeted Wesley. Then we all moved on to our next sessions. At the lunch break, Eric and I sat at a table in the large lounge area of the hotel, where we met another couple.

Eric asked his favorite question: "So, what's your poly story?"

The guy lived with his girlfriend, his ex-wife, and their two children in a house with separate areas to accommodate everyone's privacy. In this way, the two exes could more easily co-parent their children. I had heard about such households but had never met anyone living in one. He told us that he was philosophically committed to building a polycule that included his lovers and family and was constructing an addition to his house to accommodate everyone. From speaking separately with his girlfriend, I learned that they were navigating typical areas of contention in any relationship, like time management and envy.

At the time, an occasional partner of mine—called a *comet* because I saw him once a year when he came to Washington for a conference—and his wife lived in an intentional community where the members owned private living space in a small house and contributed to shared space, including a larger dining and kitchen area and an activities center for watching television or playing games together. My comet partner liked the sense of community it fostered. I did not know how prevalent such an intentional poly-focused housing complex was and had been surprised to hear there was one in Atlanta. While I did not picture myself in a poly family environment, I was heartened that they existed. Conversely, I thought that Eric, because of his communal nature when it came to relationships, would be more open to such an arrangement.

Wesley approached as Eric and I were sitting with Gina and Cooper, two other conference attendees.

"We were talking about lunch options," Eric told him. "We found an Indian place. We thought we'd take our freaky crew over there. Interested?"

"Yes, I love Indian food," Wesley said. "The timing is great since my partner is arriving after lunch."

"Can't wait to meet her," said Eric. I nodded my agreement.

Five of us piled into Gina's car. Cooper and Gina had come to the conference without partners. At a counter-service restaurant in a tiny strip mall, we sat ourselves at a square table, using plastic utensils to eat dahl and masala dishes on paper plates.

We bonded over telling our polyamory stories, tossing out terms like *poly* and *my husband's girlfriend* and *my boyfriend's wife* within earshot of the other tables. I wondered what the adjacent diners thought of us and if later they would talk about what they heard. I wanted that. I wanted *polyamory* to appear in their laptop search engines and to be a part of their dinner conversation.

Gina explained that she was dating two guys in two different states. One boyfriend knew about the other, and the other did not. In part, she was attending the conference to learn to ethically manage dating. She was concerned about being a divorced polyamorous parent and what public exposure could mean to her custody arrangement. Later at the poly conference, I attended a session called Polyamory and the Law, where the speaker shared her experience of her parents trying to gain custody of her child by attacking her as unfit merely because she was polyamorous.

Cooper had been in polyamorous relationships before, although he was not in one at that moment. He was at the conference to meet people and for a getaway from his rural home.

When it was Wesley's turn to share his poly story, he told us he had two local partners. He had met Piper when they were both married to other people. He and Piper dated monogamously after leaving their marriages. During a relationship hiatus from Piper, Wesley met Claire and learned more about polyamory. He found that polyamory philosophy fit who he was. When he and Piper talked about reuniting, he told her that he identified as polyamorous, so their renewed relationship would need to accommodate that.

Piper found that polyamory made sense to her as well. For a while, Wesley dated both Piper and Claire. I later learned that Wesley and Claire were having difficulties. Soon after the poly conference, they broke up.

After the post-lunch conference session, Eric chatted with some attendees and perused the merchandise table, which consisted mainly of polyamory-themed books, T-shirts, and stickers, leaving Wesley and me to get better acquainted. I thought I detected a flirty vibe, and just as I was about to say something about the attraction, Piper walked up. She must have sensed the intimacy in our body language because after Wesley introduced us, she excused herself. Wesley and I continued our conversation while she picked up her registration materials.

I didn't know what to make of Piper's tone. She seemed to intuit something between us before we had progressed to voicing it ourselves, and then she withdrew with a suddenness that I feared was jealousy. Even two years after my breakup with Hank, memories of Sylvia shaded my world. At that juncture, it had been five months since I had taken Hank out for a birthday dinner—I know, I know, ill-advised—and Sylvia had attacked him when he came home, broken their TV, threatened to stalk me at my workplace, and messaged me to stay away from Hank. I realized that I was getting ahead of myself with Wesley and Piper, but the hairs on the back of my neck stood up just a bit higher.

After Piper headed to the registration tables, I steeled myself and said, "Wesley, I'm attracted to you, if that's something you want to pursue."

"I feel the same," he said, grinning. "Piper just got here, and I want to connect with her and see how she is doing. Let's talk a little later?"

"Oh, of course!" I said, flushed. "No rush."

Wesley seemed rational and sensitive to others' feelings and emotions, a poster child for emotional intelligence, which I found calming. He was not new to marriage and relationships. While he might have been newer to polyamory than Eric and me, I sensed a centeredness about him that made me trust him. I hoped that we could get to know each other better over the weekend.

Eric consulted the schedule. "What looks good to you for the afternoon session? I'm thinking Ballroom A for 'Managing Jealousy.'"

I pulled Eric close and whispered, "I told Wesley I was attracted to him, and he said he was interested in me, too."

"Really?!" Eric said with feigned shock. "I could see he was into you. Good for you for speaking up."

"It's hard for me to make the first move," I said. "You know that."

"I do. That's why I invited him to lunch *and* gave you space to talk after lunch. He seems like a good guy. Fit and smart—just your type. I'm happy for you."

"He's going to talk to Piper. She seemed *your* type—curvy and vivacious," I said.

"Yes, indeed. I see potential." We kissed and parted to attend different sessions.

When the dinner break was upon us, we assembled a group, which included Piper and Wesley, and headed to a nearby chain restaurant. When I say "we," it was primarily Eric's extroverted and high-functioning planning personality that rallied us, quickly calculating who would likely be fun and interesting. He was biased toward action. I had always found his competence a heady aphrodisiac.

The restaurant was Saturday-night busy. The wait for a table gave me time to talk with Piper as we sipped drinks at the bar. While any earlier frostiness seemed to have melted, I was still Sylvia-triggered sensitive to signs of over-possessiveness. Piper told me about her prior marriage and that she had embraced polyamory after talking to Wesley and reading more about it. She came across as self-assured and pleasant, open and honest. I felt the tension in my body ease.

Eric and Wesley waited with us at the bar. We all talked, learning more about each other. Piper laughed easily and exhibited bracing honesty as she told stories of getting her tattoos, losing weight after her divorce, and her recent journey to become a certified mindfulness instructor.

Eric, per usual, was positive and extroverted. I think he was also trying to support my interest in Wesley by being friendly to both Piper and Wesley, not that it was hard to do. From his smile and jokes, I could see that Eric was enjoying their company.

After dinner, there was a brief evening program at the hotel, followed by a happy hour, but the night was unscheduled, so attendees could mingle and pursue their own desires. I checked in with Eric.

"What do you think about Piper and Wesley?"

"Piper is fun, and I can see why you like Wesley. He's a good guy," he said. "I'm open to something happening."

Piper and Wesley were sitting on a sofa in the hotel's open lounge area with their drinks. Eric squeezed in next to Piper, and I sat between Piper and Wesley, so that the guys were the bookends on a small sofa that was not meant to hold four butts. Our limbs overlapped, and we exchanged tipsy banter. We talked to other conference attendees who were sitting in the chairs surrounding the coffee table in front of our sofa. We got some smirks and raised eyebrows, but I felt them thinking, *Look at those pervs in a poly pile. Cool.*

Hooking up poly style is not all that different from hooking up single. There can be what seems like a never-ending period of awkward conversation and innuendo until someone finally kisses. Being the rather impatient person that I am, especially when it was clear to everyone who walked past us that we were into each other, I kissed Wesley. Then Eric kissed Piper.

Once that ice was broken, and we all seemed to have enjoyed the experience, we agreed to go to our hotel room.

As I had learned from swinging, when four people get together, the challenges to effective communication and the risk of hurt feelings increase exponentially. Throw two couples together who had just met, add sex and relationship anxieties, and there we were.

We four settled on the sofa and floor of the living room of our suite and practiced our *safer sex elevator speeches*, so-called because they are short enough to be given in the space of an elevator ride. The speech was designed to facilitate expressing interest in sex, addressing sexually transmitted infection (STI) test results and status, and discussing participants' wants and needs in bed before anyone took their clothes off. We had been introduced to the safer sex elevator speech concept at the conference that morning by sex-positive educator Reid Mihalko.* *Sex positivity* is a way of approaching sex with an understanding that sexuality is a healthy, shame-free, and integral part of humans and is fostered by honest communication and healthy relationships.

Nervous and excited, I was keen to get my speech over with, so I said I'd go first. As instructed by the speech protocol, I began with when I was last tested for STIs and reported any potential deal-killers—infections or conditions that

* For more on the Safer Sex Elevator Speech, see http://reidaboutsex.com/safer-sex-elevator-speech-on-the-third-date-when-to-bring-this-up/.

could take a particular type of sexual contact off the table, depending on risk tolerances of all involved.

"I was tested two months ago and everything came back clean. I don't have any conditions or infections," I said. "I try to get tested twice a year, unless there's a reason to test more often."

"Not 'clean.' Say 'negative.'" Wesley said, nudging me playfully. "Clean implies that an STI is dirty, so we say 'positive' or 'negative' test results. These days, most STIs are easily treatable."

"Right. Thanks for the reminder," I said. "As for protection, Eric and I use condoms with other partners, but not with each other. We are fluid-bonded. I don't need gloves or dental dams or any other barriers."

"Natalie, when you said you were tested, what tests did you have?" Wesley asked.

"I had a typical panel, I guess," I said, listing the ones I remembered.

"There is no typical panel. I keep mine on a spreadsheet on my phone, so I know the exact ones," Wesley said. "But I am a nerd that way."

"Nerds are hot," I teased.

Wesley smiled.

"Now that the unglamorous stuff is out of the way, we are supposed to talk about the fun stuff," I said.

This is where I was specific about what lit my fire and what left me cold. I was relieved to have the excuse of a checklist to be blunt about sex while I was upright and lucid, rather than trying to maneuver my body under his touch in the heat of the moment, using literal body language I hoped he could decipher. What a game-changer it was to say, "Don't waste your time doing this thing because it does nothing for me, but please, please do this other thing because it drives me wild." Wesley and Piper could see Eric smiling as I gave my pitch. These were lessons in my body he had learned years ago.

"Listen to her, brother," Eric chimed in. "She is telling you like it is."

I was looking forward to hearing from Wesley. What turned him on? I realized that I hadn't given intentional consideration to my male partners' likes and dislikes in bed until I was confronted with speaking of mine. I was guilty of assuming most penises worked the same.

Consulting the notes on my phone, I saw that the next item was a catch-all opportunity to add anything else I thought a new partner would need to know. I didn't have any triggers or past trauma that warranted a warning, but there was an item I had never voiced before. Here was my chance.

"I am cool with some talking during sex, whatever you're comfortable with, but I don't like to be called slut or a whore," I said. I felt weird saying that out loud in front of not only Wesley, to whom my comment was directed, but also Eric and Piper. Eric would never call me that, but some guys did. No shame if being called a good little slut is your thing. It just wasn't mine. Piper quietly sat outside of my direct line of sight.

Wesley nodded. "That's all I have," I said. Then, per the script, I asked Wesley, "How about you?" Whew, I was done. After the initial awkwardness of giving the speech for the first time, I felt unburdened and relaxed, having set the stage for maximum pleasure.

Wesley gave his speech, followed by Piper and Eric. Beyond condoms, there were no barriers needed. When I heard Piper share a trigger based on her history, I was grateful she had a safe space to take precautions to protect herself physically and emotionally. When everyone had spoken their piece, there were smiles all around as we moved to the king-sized bed.

Wesley and I occupied one side of the bed. Eric and Piper were on the other. Our limbs and fingers may have brushed our regular partners and our new metamours occasionally, but we were focused on exploring connections with our new partners.

It was past midnight when we finished fooling around, so Wesley and Piper stayed over, all four of us in one bed. Wesley spooned me the whole night. That was new to me. I tended to sleep with more space between me and my partner, as in at least some space.

No big deal, I figured. I could adjust for one night. It felt nice to be wrapped in Wesley's long arms, his knees against the backs of my knees, his nose nuzzling my neck. I was exhausted and slept like the dead, facing the wall. Eric and Piper slept on their half of the bed.

I learned in the morning that Piper had left the bed to sleep on the couch, where Eric had found her tearful.

"What's wrong, Piper?" Eric had asked.

"Wesley and I always sleep like spoons. It's hard to see him do that with Natalie. It made me feel estranged from him. And jealous."

"I understand. You know he cares for you, and tomorrow you both can talk about it."

Then Eric found other ways to comfort her.

In the morning, Piper talked to Wesley, and they had some time together alone to reconnect.

My tingling Spidey sense about Piper had not been wrong, but it had not been completely right either. She was not Sylvia. She did not lash out at me or blame me. She was dealing with her feelings the best she could. I didn't think there would be an enduring problem with Wesley connecting with me, if indeed that ever happened again, since we lived in different cities.

Piper was emotive, but she was also honest, and she and Wesley moved forward. Sometimes, a person just needs reassurance that they matter, especially when confronted with a shiny new thing. (That was *me* in this scenario—don't you dare laugh.) I understood. I'd been there. I was impressed that Piper had so effectively handled her arc from upset to calm. Eric's steadiness and empathy had helped that process, and I was grateful.

At that point in my poly life with Eric, I had seen him with enough women that I felt more compersion than jealousy. I was happy that he and Piper had connected. I was relieved that we both had sparked with both halves of the couple.

Eric and I afforded our new friends their space, maintaining some physical distance on Sunday during the conference's closing ceremony. We exchanged contact information and extended mutual invitations to visit. As it happened, about six weeks later, Piper and Wesley were driving up I-95, literally passing our house, during my birthday weekend, where the living room disco lights that Eric had lovingly installed for me would be working overtime at our dance party.

They stayed the weekend, and it was lovely. After fooling around, we cuddled on the sofa watching *Grosse Point Blank* under a blanket and ordered takeout food. At our house party, Piper and Wesley retreated into a couple's bubble while I danced my ass off, gabbed with friends, and reconnected with Felix, who surprised me by coming to the party. My sister Julia flew in for an unexpected appearance on my birthday that touched me deeply.

Leah, Eric's girlfriend of about two years by that time, was at the party. My former metamour and still friend Winnie, and her husband, my former partner Lee, also made it. They brought their new partner, Jinx, whom both Winnie and Lee were gaga over. Together, they formed a *throuple* or *triad,* where each of the three partners had intimate relations with the other, either independently or together.

I saw no jealousy in the room. I had been a little worried that Wesley and Piper would feel abandoned as I played hostess to several dozen party guests, but I was delighted to see that they were happily occupied on and off the dance floor. I think that after the four of us had spent so much concentrated time together for the prior thirty-six hours, they enjoyed the space to be a couple. I know that Eric and I savored our time as a couple, especially when we were feeling polysaturated by our other relationships. Watching them sway to the slow songs made me smile. I liked seeing their close and seemingly healthy dynamic, knowing that earlier that day Wesley and I had spent hours lounging in my bed, talking about kids, relationships, and just about everything with the ease of old friends, while Eric was in the guest room with Piper.

When Piper and Wesley got back on the road, they left me with two birthday gifts. Piper gave me a gorgeous wool scarf in magenta and black, two of my favorite colors, to replace the one I had lost at the poly conference. They also left the invaluable gift of their presence in our lives.

A week later, a box arrived at my door. This third gift from Piper was a child's delightfully flamboyant, pink, plastic foot-long wand, decorated with feathers and topped with a faux ruby heart. When shaken gently, it lit up and emitted magical, fairy-like sounds. The wand was a nod to our giggling conversation about queens and princesses as our foursome snuggled on the couch. I immediately dashed off a handwritten note to thank her.

Not only did I enjoy Wesley's company, but Piper and Eric got along, effortlessly swapping innuendos or ass slaps, and Piper and I were in a good place. I felt triply blessed.

Six months after my birthday, I loaned the wand to Leah during her birthday celebration at our house, passing the wand from one metamour to another. That, friends, is what poly podcaster Cunning Minx would have called a happy poly moment.*

Eric and Piper maintained a long-distance relationship of sorts. She invited him to a local event, and he spent the weekend with her. I was invited to keep Wesley company, but my work got in the way. On another occasion, Wesley was passing through my city without Piper. We had a hot reconnection tryst before he drove the rest of the way home. Seeing Wesley was a pleasant respite with no drama, no worries.

The months went by, and Wesley and I texted about getting together again if either of us was in the other's city. It dawned on me that we did not live that far away, and with Will away at college, my schedule was more flexible. Why not go see Wesley for a weekend? Eric and I would drive together, and once we arrived, we would split up so Eric could spend time with Piper while I was with Wesley, and the four of us could hang out if we wanted.

As the scheduled weekend approached, I realized that I preferred to reconnect with Wesley without Eric along. I was reticent to tell Eric because I felt selfish. However, the more we discussed logistics, the more difficult meshing everyone's schedules became. Piper was taking meditation classes, so she would only be available during the evenings. That left Eric on his own or third-wheeling with me and Wesley. As much as I adored my husband, I wanted time to connect with Wesley.

Eric had his weekend with Piper earlier in the summer, when I had to work. I wanted the opportunity to explore what was between Wesley and me, one-on-one. I also wanted Eric to understand that without me having to own up to it.

I am not a mind reader, Natalie, I heard Eric say in my inner dialogue.

I wanted him to realize that I had experienced only a single weekend with a lover in the seven years we had been polyamorous. That was the trip to New

---

* On her *Polyamory Weekly* podcasts, the host relayed Happy Poly Moments from her audience. Some of my moments aired over the years, including my retelling of when Marianne left a casserole in our fridge after my father died. It never failed to overjoy Eric to hear those moments on air.

York City with Hank, and we broke up a week after we came back. It had been hell to get the trip approved by Sylvia, who had groused about the timing of our three-night escape.

Admittedly, my lack of time away with my partners was not Eric's fault. He encouraged me to enjoy our open marriage and all the fun I could stand. However, when Will was too young to be left alone, Eric's trips were facilitated by my staying home with our son. More than one kink camp, weekend trips to the shore or the mountains, and a week in Europe with Lorraine were the times I stayed with Will. This was also true before our marriage was open, and Eric traveled alone for music festivals, domestically and abroad.

Eric had spent two weeks away with Leah at Pennsic just a couple of months earlier. I needed Natalie time to visit my lover. His multiple trips with his girlfriends compared jarringly to my single trip with Hank.

But I resisted whining about past inequities and told Eric I preferred a weekend alone with Wesley. Eric agreed wholeheartedly, especially since the timing of the weekend away did not work well for him and Piper. I cheered silently. I would finally get to see what a weekend with my lover could be like, one that a put-upon metamour had not grudgingly sanctioned.

I opted to take the train from Union Station. I hadn't seen Wesley in a few months, and I felt the flutter of anticipation build as the train wound from DC to my out-of-town lover. Wesley and I had been trading gushy messages full of hearts and smiling emojis for weeks, like adolescents separated by respective summer camps, counting the days until school started so we could hold hands in the hallways and eat lunch together.

More often than I would have expected, polyamory made me feel like a teenager. I wiped my sweaty palms on my jeans that Friday evening as the train pulled into the station. Wesley and I had made no specific plans. We would let the evening unfold.

I liked new people in my life to choose restaurants and outings, even steer the conversation, because it let me learn about them, what they liked, and what mattered to them. I wanted to relax and let the weekend flow. I did not want to be responsible for planning. I sensed that with Wesley, I could be me, messy morning hair, makeup-free face, impolitic attitudes, and all.

When I walked up the steps from the train platform and reached the cavernous station proper, there was Wesley, beaming at me. I beamed back. He scooped me up in his long arms and squeezed me against his chest. I had to stand on tiptoes to meet his lips. I mainly kissed the teeth of his smile, and that made me smile too. Our teeth clicked and we laughed. He put his arm around my waist and pulled me in close as we walked to the station counter to store my bag before exiting the station to find dinner in the city. This was his town, so he led the way.

He kept grinning at me. I was flattered, basking in his happiness, while also a bit befuddled that I sparked such joy. Part of my skepticism was because Wesley was a dozen years younger than me. *What does he see in an old lady like me?* tugged at the edge of my bliss. Gratefully, the internal chorus of my girlfriends and my husband broke through my self-doubt. *Of course he is happy to be with you. You are smart, attractive, and fun to be around. Don't sell yourself short. He's lucky and he knows it.* I let myself accept his warmth, and I held his hand tighter.

I felt free. I had never found a staycation relaxing. I liked to travel for work, to be in a different place for a while where I was only responsible for myself. Eric would say that he didn't ask me to cook or shop for him or do laundry. It was just our division of labor. I liked taking care of my boys. I liked seeing them enjoy my simple meals. Even though no one would starve for the few days I was gone, I still left them precooked meals if I could, fretting that I had not left enough.

Why was I like that? Because that was what my mother did? Because that's what I thought I was supposed to do? Because my role as wife, mother, and caretaker of the house and family was one I valued? All of that, I guess. The point was that when I was away from home, I felt the tension between my shoulders ease and my step lighten as I began my weekend with a lover who seemed jubilant to see me. I was surprised I could walk in a straightish line under the influence of the heady intoxication of NRE and freedom.

Our compatibility was so effortless that I felt as if we were wandering through a misty film set where we were the main characters, and everyone else had supporting roles designed to maximize our joy. We hiked in the woods near Wesley's house, and he identified trees and plants along the trail. He showed me his carpentry workspace in the basement and the magical outer door on his fridge that slid open to reveal space for those everyday essentials like orange juice. I was impressed by both.

We made smoothies so packed with fruit and peanut butter that the blender started smoking. We walked to dinner at the neighborhood restaurant where Wesley was a regular and bantered with the waitress, who snarked about other patrons. We traded full-body massages and washed the coconut oil off each other's backs in the shower.

We talked and talked and talked. Wesley told me more about his former partner, Claire, whom he had been dating when I met him. He was having a hard time dealing with their recent breakup, and he found it awkward to talk to Piper about it because there had been friction between the two metamours. Talking to me helped him process the relationship and its ending. I listened patiently, without bias. His face often brightened when he spoke of her, recalling how she added to his life in ways that Piper did not because Claire and Piper were different.

Wasn't that one of the reasons we engaged in polyamory? It permitted us to love different people at the same time for different reasons, at different depths, and for different durations. Claire's absence left a void in Wesley's life. He was looking for a local partner to fill it, but the void remained. I was not a candidate to be the nearby full-time partner that his lost love had been, but I was happy to be part of his life for as long as we lasted.

Like me, Wesley had raised a son. Sam was almost the same age as Will. I did not meet Wesley's son that weekend, but I learned about how Wesley parented him. Listening to him talk about Sam opened the door even more to Wesley, and in turn let me talk about Will and gain Wesley's perspective. When Wesley and Will had met during his and Piper's dance party weekend visit some months earlier, they interacted easily. It made me happy when my partners and my son got along. Hank and Will were Xbox buddies, and Lee had loaned Will a set of graphic novels.

Wesley and I didn't drive anywhere during my weekend visit until I held on to his waist for the motorcycle ride to the train station. On my journey home, I couldn't think of a single way our weekend could have been better. I cherished the cocoon we shared for those two days and nights. It felt almost like a honeymoon;

we were so absorbed in each other. We agreed to see one another soon, and we did.

Two months later, we spent our Friday evening at his local poly meetup. I was touched to be invited because I knew he would introduce me to those who knew him and Piper as a couple as his out-of-town partner. Wesley preferred that term to girlfriend. I had not been in that situation before. Eric introduced Marianne as his girlfriend, but I think only Lee had ever referred to me as his girlfriend.

I wondered if it was juvenile or possessive for a middle-aged woman to want to be called someone's girlfriend or partner. I think it was not so much the label as the acknowledgment that I was connected to someone who was happy to announce it in public. Hank would not introduce me to his friends at all, much less call me his girlfriend, at least in my presence. I remember running into his friends when we were on a date. Hank talked to them and ignored me as I stood at his elbow. I could understand his introducing me as his friend rather than his partner, but to disregard me so completely made me feel tainted. I learned later that Sylvia forbade Hank from introducing me to their friends. Yes, you may roll your eyes.

Wesley was comfortable identifying as polyamorous and therefore was comfortable with the poly labels. I was his partner from out of town. Piper was his local partner. I thought of Piper as Wesley's anchor or primary partner, just as Eric was mine. Being in an environment of poly people at a poly meetup with my poly boyfriend made me feel valued. I didn't see that as juvenile. I saw it as kind and as normalizing polyamory.

Piper, Wesley, Eric, and I spent time together periodically, and we also spent time separately in our secondary partner pairs. The more time I spent with Piper, the more I liked her. Piper was older than most of Eric's other partners. She had an easy confidence and an impish way that made me grin. I liked seeing her challenge and poke Eric in the silly ways that lovers do. I wished there were fewer miles between us.

Six months after we met, Wesley and I were texting, the primary way we communicated, when he mentioned he would be traveling to India for work.

"Ooh, that sounds amazing," I gushed.

"I'm looking forward to it," he responded. "I plan to take two weeks of vacation after the work part is done to explore the country. I've never been, and since my job is paying for the airfare, I might as well get the most out of it."

"Is Piper joining you?"

"No, not this trip, but she is already making a list of things she wants me to bring back."

"Gifts are her love language," I typed back.

I hesitated. Then I typed, "If you wanted a travel buddy, I would love to see India." I added, "and I could pay my way."

I immediately wondered if I had overstepped our new relationship. I was about to backtrack when I saw the ellipses that signaled Wesley typing.

"I would like that," he responded, his message ending with a smiling emoji.

"Cool! Let me talk to Eric and get back to you?"

"Sounds good. Talk to you soon!" Wesley ended the chat with a kissing emoji.

My heart was racing, and my feet followed. I nearly tripped down the stairs to our shared office, where Eric was sitting at his computer.

"Eric," I said, "can I talk to you about something?"

He turned and looked at me. "Are you okay? You seem out of breath."

"Yes, I am more than okay." I smiled. I sat in the armchair in the corner of the room, the same armchair where Eric had sat six years earlier and proposed that we try polyamory and that he date Lorraine.

I tried to collect myself. "Wesley has a work trip to India. He's planning to travel afterward," I began. "We talked about me going with him." I studied Eric for signs of his reaction.

"India?" Eric said. "That sounds like quite an adventure."

"Doesn't it? I think so, too. How do you feel about me joining him for a week or so?"

"Natalie." Eric smiled. "You know how much I like Wesley. I trust that you'll be safe with him. He's a great guy, a smart guy. If you want to go, I say, go!"

"Really?" I exhaled.

"Of course, really," he said. "I am happy for you. Isn't this why we do poly? I have no desire to go to India, and I am happy you have this opportunity to go with a partner. I want you to have all the fun and come home full of stories to tell me."

I sat on his lap and kissed him. "Thank you, Eric. My first overseas trip with another partner! I am excited."

"I noticed," Eric said, laughing. "I like seeing you like this."

I should not have been surprised at Eric's reaction. He had never begrudged me any joy I could derive from polyamory. I also knew he was aware that I had felt shortchanged by my lack of getaways with other partners. With Will away at college, Eric agreed that I should lean into empty nest advantages. I didn't worry much about Eric being occupied while I was in India. He had his job, his goth and kink events, and his local partners, primarily Leah, to keep him company. The company of others nourished Eric. I felt better about leaving, knowing he would not be hungry.

I messaged Wesley. "Eric is fully supportive. He thinks very highly of you. Perhaps it's your excellent choice in women?"

"We do agree that you're hot, so there's that," Wesley typed.

"Is my joining you in India weird?"

"Haha. You don't mean because we have known each other less than a year, only spent two consecutive nights together a few times, and we will be with each other 24/7 for a week in another country?"

"Yeah, that."

"I'm not worried. Are you?"

"Strangely," I responded, "I'm not. I have a sense that we'll get along well. I'm looking forward to this adventure with you."

"Same!" he typed.

Over the next few months, Wesley and I traded Google Docs with links and maps of places to visit. I checked on visas and other entry requirements. Neither of us had been to India, so I was grateful when Wesley offered to handle most of the logistics and consult a travel agent. He would be working in southern India for a couple of weeks, so he would have a lay of the land by the time I arrived, having taken a solo trip north to Delhi and Jaipur. Wesley hired a driver for part of our trip and booked the hotels. I was responsible for getting myself to and from India and paying my share of the ground expenses. My travel anxiety quieted knowing my partner was competent and calm. Acts of service had always been my primary love language, and trip planning was a service I coveted. I shared the details as they developed with Eric, who, in turn, shared my excitement.

The day before my flight, I shopped the costume jewelry racks and found one more thing I needed for my trip. I bought a twenty-dollar wedding band. The diamond ring set from Eric, which I had been wearing for twenty-five years, stayed on my dresser at home, safe from thieves and loss. My hand felt naked without the rings. I was married, even when I was with Wesley, so I wore the simple band on my left hand.

On my departure date, Eric drove me to the airport. He held me close in his arms, and we kissed tenderly. His kisses calmed me.

"You and Wesley are going to have a great time. Send pictures of you smiling, and that will make my day. Don't worry, okay? I love you."

"I love you, too."

I slung on my backpack and grabbed my carry-on, waving to Eric as I walked through the sliding doors of the airport. I made a mental note to swallow the Dramamine pill in my pocket before boarding. Motion sickness had plagued me since childhood.

Twenty hours later, Wesley met me at the airport in Bengaluru, India, greeting me with an expansive smile that soothed and excited me.

Over the week, we enjoyed oil-laden massages, swam in spring-fed pools, and visited a sixteenth-century synagogue. We wandered parks, markets, and museums and bought spices cultivated from hills we climbed. My luggage smelled of cinnamon and garam masala.

Standing well over six feet tall with light brown hair and light blue eyes, Wesley was an attraction to the Indian boys who waved at him on the street, shouting and smiling to get his attention. In a local park on a Sunday afternoon, an Indian family asked us to take their photo. When Wesley accepted their phone to snap a picture, they gestured for the two of us to be in the photo. We smiled as we huddled together with the parents, two children, and grandmother, and Wesley's long arm captured the moment with a shutter click. Only after the family smiled their thanks and were on their way did I realize that we were an oddity with our light skin and Western looks. My red and black hair likely contributed to our otherness. The tourists we identified from their heads bent over map apps on their phones and squinting up at street signs appeared to be Indians, rather than international travelers.

I had never been on a safari, and it was the booking I was anticipating the most. When our nighttime excursion did not yield the animal sightings I had dreamed of from my weekly childhood viewings of *Wild Kingdom*—especially elephants!—instead of sitting in my disappointment, I mentioned it to Wesley and our driver. The driver knew of a tourist spot where we could ride and bathe elephants. Bathe elephants? I was wide-eyed.

Wesley was not interested in bathing an elephant—whatever that entailed—so he held on to my phone while I used a long-handled brush to scrub the gray folds of the gigantic but docile animal. The handler directed me to climb astride the elephant as she bowed down to accommodate me. I obliged, and the pachyderm rose with me on her back. It was as if I were outside my body and looking at myself on a large movie screen. Cue the Indiana Jones music!

I felt heady as the beast rose and I gained altitude. As I was steadying myself, an explosion of water sprayed my face. I gasped. Before I could say anything, my new bathing buddy reloaded her trunk from her water trough and doused me again. I was filled with unexpected delight as I held on to the elephant's neck and she continued to spray me with the power of a Super Soaker. I laughed and squealed like a five-year-old experiencing her first amusement park ride.

When the elephant finished bathing me, she bent her knees and lowered me to the ground. I was drenched. Then I understood why visitors were told to bring a change of clothes. Wiping water from my eyes and sputtering, I saw that Wesley was grinning from the safety of dry land.

"Look," he said, holding up my phone.

He had taken a dozen quick photos that, when viewed serially, were a stop-action flip book of the elephant spraying me as I laughed and grew progressively wetter.

"That was so much fun!" I grinned. "I'm glad we stopped here. It has been a highlight of my trip." I gave Wesley a wet kiss.

"You looked so happy up there. Wait until Eric sees these photos," Wesley said. "He's going to love them!" He had already snuck a photo of me in my bathing suit at the hotel pool and sent it to Eric, which had elicited heart and fire emojis from my husband. That my two partners seemed to harbor no jealousy in sharing me had me walking on air. That they traded snickers like frat brothers on how good I looked in a bikini made me blush.

A photograph of me on top of the elephant, her trunk raised in an S-shaped arc, the water spray frozen in the frame as it showered me, my laughter evident, served as my social media profile picture for months after our trip. It was a reminder of the joy I felt at that moment during my first overseas trip with a poly partner to a land I had never visited, with the full support of my husband.

I was intoxicated with polyamorous pleasure as I wrung out my clothes and changed before our drive down the mountains, sitting shotgun and armed with ginger root to chew to stem the unrelenting motion sickness I had suffered on the ride up in the backseat. My stomach remained calm, and my heart remained full.

Wesley told me later that our driver had asked at the start of the trip if we were married.

"Well, *I* am," I said, laughing. "What did you tell him?"

"I said we were. It seemed easier than explaining polyamory to him. You know?"

I didn't know it at the time, but the trip with Wesley would be the first of many vacations with partners, both with and without Eric, that my poly life would bring me.

22.
Morning After

I watched Adam sling his backpack over one broad shoulder. He wore his girlfriend's elastic headband to hold back his long-on-top, short-on-the-sides, sun-colored locks. He had morning hair, and so did I. Adam ambled down my front steps on impossibly long legs. I lingered for a moment at the window, sipping my coffee, appreciating his casual good looks—tall, slim, and strong-jawed. Adam would have blushed to hear me describe him this way, seemingly bashfully unaware of his intoxicating presence. He had an endearing way of rolling his amber eyes and reddening when receiving compliments, but he had to know he was model-hot.

"Thanks for having me over," he had said in the doorway as he tipped his head down and his full, soft lips found mine.

"Any time." I smiled up at him.

I was suddenly wistful. It was nine on a sunny, chilly Sunday morning. Today there was no sleeping in or cooking an unhurried breakfast. Adam's live-in girlfriend Sydney had been texting him about needing their car.

As of that morning goodbye, I had been seeing Adam for seven months, about seven months longer than I had anticipated before our first date. Adam had sent me a simple "Hi, Natalie" message on a dating site. His profile picture showed him with his clean-shaven chin propped in his long-fingered hand, looking sideways at the camera in a way both innocent and smoldering. Although I was enticed by well-chosen photos of him with his girlfriend, him with his dog, him with his nephew, and him playing soccer—no seat-belted selfies or awkwardly posed, towel-wearing, bathroom mirror reflection pictures—I wanted to read his full profile before responding.

We overlapped on some music tastes like the Rolling Stones and the Beatles. Was this guy really twenty-six? His summary was written with self-deprecation and turns of phrase like "I am living in the city and trying to convince myself that I am better than people who live in the suburbs," where it turned out he grew up with four siblings, all of them tall, thin, and fair-haired. In pictures, his family looked like a Mormon wet dream. I saw Sydney in one, like a dark spot on the sun. Her features and coloring were not dissimilar to mine.

Adam's profile ended with "Contact me if you are cool with polyamory." Well, then.

"Hey, Adam," I messaged back. "Always encouraging to see poly represent on here."

We chatted about how long we had been polyamorous.

Me: Ethically non-monogamous since 2000ish. Poly since about 2010. It kind of depends on how you count. You?

Him: Only about a year, so I am pretty new to it.

My poly-sense was tingling. Did I want to get involved with a newbie?

Me: You have to start somewhere. How's it going? Is your girlfriend into it?

Him: It's gone well so far! And yeah, she's way into it. She introduced me to the concept.

We messaged more over the next week and set up a drinks date. It was for the same night that Leah was coming over to the house to cook dinner with Eric—and me if I was around. I told Eric that my plan was a quick drink with Adam after work, and then I'd be home for dinner, but not to wait for me. I saw little chance that the date would go anywhere because of the age and hotness gap and his newness to poly, but I liked meeting poly people, and we seemed to click at least superficially.

Adam was dreamy. I could picture him on a fifty-foot-high billboard in a stark white T-shirt and faded, soft-looking blue jeans, barefoot in the sand, with his arm crooked to shield his brow against the California sun. Whatever he wanted you to buy—cologne, sunglasses, Bitcoin—you would sell your grandmother's wheelchair for the cash to get it. I was flattered that he wanted to meet me. I also had a date planned for the following weekend with a fortysomething guy from the same dating site. My odds were not on Adam.

I arrived a few minutes early at the bar Adam had suggested. It was a classy little underground spot called Off the Record with a circular bar in the center of the room. I walked past the hotel doorman to the back of the first floor and down a narrow flight of steps. I looked around and realized Adam had not arrived yet. The bar was nearly empty, early on a weeknight.

I debated whether to sit at the bar, but the thought made me uncomfortable. If I ordered a drink and Adam didn't show up, I was a sad middle-aged woman on a barstool. You might say, as Eric would, "Natalie, what century do you think this is? There is nothing wrong with a woman sitting alone at a bar ordering a drink." Maybe so, but I was not that woman.

As I walked toward the restrooms, I saw, through a full-length window, a guy standing outside trying to open an exterior door to the hallway leading to the bar. The door didn't budge, and he peered in briefly. Ah, he didn't know you had to enter from upstairs. I had almost made the same mistake. *That looks like Adam*, I thought. I could have tried to open the door for him, but before I made a decision, he turned away, realizing his error.

I retreated to the bathroom to fiddle with my makeup long enough for him to walk upstairs to the hotel's front entrance, take the stairs down to the bar, and find a seat. When I entered the bar, he was sitting on a barstool facing the entrance, his phone in his hand, likely about to text me. I suppressed a smile and tried to focus on good posture. Head high, tummy in. I had chosen a summer dress with a deep V-neck and a hem that fell above my knee.

We talked about our poly lives, family, politics, and movies we had seen. I was surprised at how easily the conversation flowed without the usual first-date pretension of projecting how clever or well-connected we were. Adam admitted that he had tried to enter from a locked door. I liked his honesty.

"I felt pretty silly." He grinned. "I forgot you couldn't get in that way."

"It's tricky," I said. "I had to ask the doorman how to get down here the first time I came here. This place is like a secret 1920s speakeasy."

"I know, right?" Adam said. "Easier to have a private conversation."

When our drink glasses were almost empty, the bartender asked if we wanted another round. I looked at Adam, whose nod indicated he was ready for beer number two. I said, "Not quite yet." I excused myself to the restroom. I texted Eric, worried that I had made plans to come home for dinner, but that I was not ready to leave Adam.

Me: I am having a good time and want to stay for a second drink, but I don't want to hold you and Leah up for dinner.

Eric: Enjoy yourself! Don't worry. There will be food for you whenever you get home.

Me: Thanks ☺

I slid back onto my barstool and ordered another drink. Adam and I talked about the latest political outrage being debated on the TV screen over the bar. We glanced at the other patrons.

"See those two guys and the girl? They both want her, but she's into the waitress, and neither guy has a clue," I said.

"What about that table? Are they from out of town, or just a girls' night out? So much giggling," Eric said, joining in my game.

I ate an alarming number of peanuts and wasabi peas from the dish on the bar; even more when Adam was in the restroom. I hadn't eaten dinner, and it was way past now. Adam ate nothing.

Adam leaned in so close I could feel the warmth of his taut body. He breathed, "I really want to kiss you."

I felt tingly and maybe a little lightheaded. "Go ahead."

He kissed me gently, right in front of the bartender. My temperature rose.

Then I thought, *I am old enough to be his mother. Are we creeping out anyone here, and, if so, how much do I care?*

We walked out of the bar together.

"You're tall," I said glancing up at him. He had twelve inches on me.

His shoulders shrugged an inch as if to say, "Yeah, I hear that a lot," but he was too polite to say it out loud.

We came to the point where our homeward paths parted. I stood on my toes, and we kissed in earnest, our torsos touching, hands in hair, tongue finding tongue. We were standing on a city street corner at nearly ten at night, each of us wishing we could duck into the bushes, if there had been any, and commit a Class 2 misdemeanor; or maybe that was just me.

The weekend following our date, Adam and I got together at my house. Not surprisingly, we synced immediately and enjoyed a steamy connection before he left down my front steps to go home to Sydney.

Wesley and I messaged the next week, catching up. He had been to a retreat and had hooked up with someone quite a bit younger.

"Go, you," I said. "I'm glad you had a good time. I thought you all slept in some kind of bunkhouse. How did that work?"

"I paid extra for my own room. Totally worth it." I could hear the grin in his typing.

"I met someone new. He's younger, too," I said.

"Oh yeah, how old? Is he 18?" he asked.

"He's over 21, thanks."

"Is he 22?"

"Ha. Ha. No." I was not amused.

"Don't keep me guessing."

"Umm."

"I'll start making it awkward," he typed.

"Start?!"

"Will plus 3," he typed.

Yeah, he just made it weird.

I paused.

"Plus 6," I typed.

"Damn, you go girl!!!"

"Okay, okay, enough."

"Color me envious," Wesley typed with a winky face.

A few months later, Eric and I hosted a dance party at the house. Adam came with Sydney.

"Is everyone here poly?" Adam asked.

"Everyone? No," I said.

I surveyed the room from our seated vantage point and explained how folks identified. Of thirty people, four couples were poly, including Eric and me. One couple were sometime swingers. One couple fell into the kinky camp. There were a few former lovers of mine and one current girlfriend of Eric's, who arrived with her live-in boyfriend. The rest were aware of my relationship dynamic, I assumed, but were not engaged in it themselves.

I didn't broadcast my polyamory at our parties, but I might mention aloud that "while Eric [or I] was on a date . . ." Several couples at the party were dating monogamously. I had also invited some unattached friends with whom I felt comfortable being my complete self. By the time of that particular dance party, Will was in college and knew his parents were polyamorous. We didn't go out of our way to tag our guests with relationship labels. Will knew our guests as our friends, but he might also be present when Eric or I were more familiar with a partner, such as a kiss on the lips hello or goodbye. I noticed that Will was dancing with one of my former metamours. Will had some moves, but then, so did his dad.

23.

Finding Friends in All the Weird Places

Eric smiled. "Camping!"

I winced. "You mean in a tent?"

I hadn't slept in a tent since fifth-grade Girl Scouts. It was not that I actively disliked camping, but I did not come from a camping family. We were a reading family. Dad would sit on one end of the sofa and read British mysteries and engineering journals—his glasses off. Mom would park in the La-Z-Boy, her reading glasses on a chain around her neck, with a Stephen King novel or *TIME* magazine. After a coveted trip to the library, I could easily spend a weekend afternoon escaping into *The Island of the Blue Dolphins*, Narnia, the Rue Morgue, a biography of Thomas Edison, or, later, a dozen fictional New England towns, courtesy of Messieurs Irving and King.

We would emerge from our respective other worlds to gather for meals, to run errands, or for father-daughter sessions on how to throw a spiral or return a serve with topspin.

"You don't want to throw like a girl, Natalie."

Twelve-year-old me rolled my eyes. "Dad, I *am* a girl."

By the time I met Eric in college, he had camped his fill with the Army National Guard, so he did not suggest camping until he did. Eric's camping proposal to me was connected to an adult camp we had attended twice before. We had participated in some of the kink offerings, but we had stayed in cabins. We called the BDSM event "kink camp" as a shorthand. Over the years of exploring non-monogamy, from swinging to polyamory, I learned that alternative lifestyle communities—be they burners, non-monogamists, goths, kinksters, or situational sadists—had a large overlap. Kink events routinely included classes about polyamory in addition to workshops demonstrating fisting or how to tie rope harnesses to suspend an adult from a metal frame. I gravitated toward the classes on relationships and rope. Eric usually attended those classes with me, but I would bow out of the single tail whip demos and the Orgies for Beginners classes. Workshops on navigating kink events with multiple partners or effectively communicating with partners and metamours were classes I both attended and taught.

The event organizers spent admirable energy erecting metal scaffolding to support BDSM equipment in a structure that served as a dungeon outfitted with the typical accoutrements such as spanking benches and large St. Andrews crosses, where a *bottom* could be cuffed or tied to the eight-foot wooden X while being consensually subjected to impact play by a *top*. *Impact play* could be anything from soft leather floggers brushing a bottom to stingy riding crops leaving red trails on backsides and legs that would turn to yellow and blue bruises that bottoms wore with pride.

Inside the dungeon were tables for *wax play*, where skin-safe wax was dripped carefully onto flesh, and for *medical play*, where as many as dozens of hollow, single-use, sterilized needles were inserted under the skin in patterns or holding colorful ribbons that could be tied up in bows. I once witnessed rows of needles laced with string that the top strummed as if the bottom was a musical instrument. The possibilities were infinite.

Camp personnel outfitted the three large tents that made up the "Shag Shack" with multiple futons and sex stations—tables that held lube, condoms, rubber gloves, wipes, tissues, chucks (thin disposable bed pads), and paper towels. Under the tables, large plastic bins labeled "clean" and "dirty" held sheets. I relished the Shag Shack for its cool breezes amid the summer heat, a welcome respite from sex in an enclosed two-person tent or a stifling cabin of strangers.

Consent culture was paramount at BDSM events, meaning that explicit, verbal consent was a prerequisite for any physical touching, sexual activity, or other BDSM engagement, especially power exchanges. Event staff could include a consent counselor as a resource or referee when a party to an interaction felt they experienced a *consent violation*, experiencing actions they did not consent to.

Often these counselors were licensed therapists. At a minimum, a *play space monitor* (PM) was present on the dungeon floor for logistical safety and emergencies.

While I witnessed many scenes, I participated in very few. I liked the eroticism, but not the pain. The BDSM world was more Eric's than mine. His attraction to the kink scene was primarily as a top. He was a natural leader, planner, and executor of scenes. I thought of competence as being one of his love languages. He didn't derive sadistic pleasure from another's pain, but he enjoyed meeting the needs of his partners.

He learned shibari, the Japanese art of the decorative tying of partners, including me. I particularly liked when he tied me with vibrant ropes of red and gold. He installed hard points in our basement ceiling strong enough to hold his partners while suspended. He raided our garage tools and used his carpentry skills and his military discount at Home Depot to buy wood to make paddles for his other partners.

If pressed to categorize myself, I would have said I was a lazy, decorative bottom and a periodic top. I might top during sex with a partner new to kink, playing the naughty nurse who administers to the bed-bound, blindfolded patient. I am not admitting that there is anything in my closet akin to a white vinyl snap-up mini-dress with a red collar, nurse's cap, white thigh-highs, crimson pumps, and a working stethoscope. Nope.

Eric had pitched a tent at the kink camp twice before with his girlfriend, Leah, whose nesting partner, Ronan, also attended the event. Leah would split her nights between Eric's tent and Ronan's. I had been relieved that Leah was game to attend the kink camp. Her BDSM tastes meshed with Eric's. She liked being displayed and watched, and Eric liked to show her off. She could be naked on a futon in the Shag Shack or in the dungeon dressed only in glittery, silver platform stripper heels—remnants from her dancer days—with her wrists bound by rope and her ass exposed for flogging or paddling, her lipsticked mouth issuing squeals of delight and gasps of pain in roughly equal measure.

Eric and I might engage in some light fun in the dungeon, but it was not my fun of choice since I was not masochistic, flinching from all but the slightest pain. Eric might use a knife to cut a dress off my body while I stood on my tiptoes, my hands bound over my head with a rope knotted to a point above as I turned and twisted out of his reach. Those episodes were mainly for Eric to "show off my sexy wife." Nonetheless, I did delight in his mischievous joy and the feel of his hands on my body.

I discovered that, as a change of pace, I enjoyed the sex swing, a canvas hammock dangling from its four corners on chains to the ceiling of the dungeon. I reclined in the swing, holding on to the chains within grasp of each hand, my legs in the air or my feet anchored on the chains. Eric stood between my legs. The height of the swing was adjustable to facilitate sex play. From my perspective, I could not see anyone but Eric. Since being watched distracted me, pulling me out of the shared experience with Eric, this position worked for me. It also satisfied Eric's exhibitionist penchant.

Before we arrived at the campsite, Eric explained that we would sleep in a tent without electricity, but we would have access to showers and bathrooms in the cabins and hot food in the dining hall.

Despite the mosquitoes biting us as we slept, and my back aching for a better sleeping mat, I discovered that I liked tent camping in our little corner of the property, away from the din of the partying. I watched with wonder as daddy longlegs clung to the inside of the tent, glistening in the backlight of the morning sun. At night, we huddled in blankets around a fire and made s'mores with friends. We were far enough from the main area that the late-night lights were not distracting, and constellations were visible in the blackness overhead. I even peed at the edge of the tree line a few times during the night to avoid the dark trek to the shared toilets. Look at me, roughing it.

The five-day event boasted classes and planned activities as well as swimming (no suits required!), dancing, and drinking. Eric and I hosted our first polyamory mixer, where dozens of campers traded stories, made new friends, and rekindled old acquaintances.

Campers volunteered to provide services that matched their kinks. A middle-aged guy with a foot fetish gave pedicures. A thirtysomething offered to insert needles just under the skin to produce an endorphin rush or for the decorative art of threading vibrant ribbons in a zigzag pattern on the bottom's back, simulating a laced corset. The camp message board might have this post: "I am looking to top for needle play. If you want to bottom, sign up at Cabin 4."

I signed up for a massage offered by a service-oriented camper. This was a leap of faith for me because I was ill at ease having strangers, including professional masseurs, knead my muscles. I was most comfortable with Eric, who knew my body's aches and was able to soothe my stresses and pains better in ten minutes than anyone else could in an hour.

My camp massage lasted four hours. No happy endings, just all-over, feel-good body rubs. We chatted the entire time. He had lived a nomadic life, traveling throughout the United States. By the end of the massage, I felt like I had known him for years and invited him for Thanksgiving. It's possible that the half-dose of acid—my first hit ever—might have been a factor.

After being face down for so long on the massage table, I was a little unsteady on my feet. It was midnight when I walked to the dining hall to hydrate. As I pushed a plastic cup under the water dispenser, I saw Violet, Zoey, and Dennis sitting at a long dining table in the otherwise deserted cafeteria.

The three friends who identified as polyamorous had flown in from out of state. Violet and Dennis were engaged. The exact nature of Violet and Zoey's connection was unclear to me, although I could see from their joking and nudging that they were close—whether platonic girlfriends, kink partners, or something else.

Earlier in the day, Zoey had stopped me as I walked past the lively voices of the Queer Mixer. Over the upbeat music, I heard her say, "Dennis is into you, in case you didn't know." She smiled a secret smile. I tried not to look as baffled as I felt and said, "No, I didn't. Thanks."

The five of us had been friendly since the first day, often eating together in the mess hall, and greeting each other with waves and smiles around camp, but those three had specific kink scenes planned for the weekend, and Eric and I had local friends we were hanging with and hooking up with. I had not sensed that Dennis was attracted to me other than as a friend. Was I still that clueless about men?

Leah had come to camp by herself that year, opting to pitch her tent on the opposite side of camp from us. We had welcomed her to camp next to us, but she chose to keep her own space. I understood her desire to center. Camp was an opportunity to be as introverted or extroverted as you chose, and Leah wanted to nurture her quieter side. She and Eric would still have time together. I didn't have a partner other than Eric with me at camp. That was okay for a while, but sometimes I got in a funk if I felt left out of the fun.

"Sometimes?" Eric might say with a loving, been-there, lived-it smirk. I could turn petulant. It was not an attractive look.

That day I had been feeling that polyamory was working a helluva lot better for Eric than for me. I had attended some interesting classes on relationships and rope bondage for sex, but I had not connected physically with anyone, nor had I made plans to. Walking across camp in search of someone to talk to or something to do that afternoon, I had strolled by the Shag Shack, the futon-filled space under a tent canopy that was one of my favorite play spots.

Eric was with Leah and a woman I didn't recognize on one of the futons, reclining in a postcoital tangle. While I knew they would have welcomed a hello from me and been happy for me to sit on the edge of the bed or even join them, it was not my thing, and I was in a churlish mood that I knew I should not impose on them.

My ill humor was because I had thought I would be able to reconnect with an old lover, CJ, but that had fizzled. He was new to open relationships and to kink, but his girlfriend made the flight plans, and he was not cleared for a solo takeoff with me. They were *situationally polyamorous.* If they were at an event away from home, playing with others was an exciting diversion. She liked watching him with other women in scenarios she planned. For him to have private time with someone was, I learned, not as much a part of their kind of polyamory as it was mine.

CJ was approved to participate in a sensory deprivation group activity I had planned, where I was blindfolded in the company of three guys I had chosen—Eric, CJ, and another man I had sex with previously, so I knew I had a connection with them and I trusted them. CJ's girlfriend watched and thoroughly enjoyed herself, according to Eric's account to me afterward. My blindfold kept me from seeing her masturbatory climaxes, but I had no earplugs to block her moans.

I concluded that while it was an interesting experiment conducted on a queen-sized mattress in a corner of a grassy area, awash in thumpy music from the dungeon and campers' voices from the pool, I felt sensory overload from the bodies on and inside mine, their aromas, tastes, and sounds. The mini-gang bang confirmed that my preference was to focus one-on-one. Polyamory meant more than one intimate relationship, but for me, it usually meant sexual intimacy with one person at a time.

On that, Eric and I differed. He was a "*moresomes* are better than threesomes are better than twosomes!" kind of sexual being. I preferred the term moresomes to *orgies*. One of the aspects of polyamory that I valued was the focus on individual connections, rather than being part of a group experience. I had tried group sex when we were in our swinging phase, and I was happy to subcontract that out to partners of Eric who enjoyed it more than I did.

In the dining hall, I filled my cup with water and greeted Zoey, Violet, and Dennis. Following an intense BDSM scene in the dungeon, Zoey was trying to re-center herself, and Violet was comforting and hydrating her as part of *aftercare.*

I sat down next to Dennis. Violet ushered Zoey back to their cabin to continue the decompression, leaving me and Dennis alone in the brightly lit hall. It was clear that they were giving us space, which telegraphed to me that Zoey *and* Violet thought Dennis liked me, even if I couldn't see it.

I was awful at flirting. Coming of age in the '80s, I expected the guy to make the first move. I had to retrain myself to be *biased toward action*, a term Eric liked to use. When I groused that men rarely approached me—was my affect too flat?—Eric told me that men's fear of being seen as creepy could make them hesitate, absent unmistakable signs of interest. Flashing neon ones were especially helpful. Keeping this in mind, as well as what Zoey told me, and prompted by a smile that reached Dennis's sparkling eyes—was he micro-flirting?—I held his face and kissed him. When he didn't turn and spit, I took that as a good sign. He kissed me back.

With my face almost touching his, I asked, "Do you want to go to the Shag Shack?" I barely got the words out before he grinned and nodded. "Yes."

I took his hand, and we walked to the open-air tents. After a brief exchange of recent STI results and agreement on the need for condoms, we explored each other's bodies. Dennis was flush and happy as he praised my skills in bringing him to climax in a way that was atypical for him. I was equally effusive in how he led me to the edge, teasing me to make my pleasure sweeter. We lay on our sides facing each other and talked in hushed tones as a breeze wafted between the tent flaps and over our damp bodies.

Dennis told me he had wanted to approach me several times and was glad I had taken the initiative. He told me about his relationship with Violet, a professional dominatrix, and their long-term friendship with Zoey. He showed me a pendant around his neck, similar to one Violet wore. They were to be married within the year. He brightened when he talked about his beloved and their courtship. He shared intimacies with me without shame or discomfort. We held each other and enjoyed the moonlit sky as the night air cooled us.

The fates being in my favor, not only did Dennis live near where I traveled for work, but he was in my neighborhood a few times a year for his job. A month after camp, he had a hotel room a mile from my house, and we spent two nights together. I took him to a bar where a deejay friend was spinning, and he met my friend Trisha. He was engaging and polite. When Dennis was getting drinks, Trisha whispered, "He's cute. And smart. Well done, girl."

We held hands and walked past a pizza joint. It was where I had devoured a slice on my first date with Hank almost six years before. As Dennis and I talked about favorite desserts, the universe spoke. Across the street, a blue, neon, moon-shaped sign I had never seen before beckoned. We climbed the steps to Celestial Sweets, a newly opened cookie and ice cream shop. I laughed, recalling Hank's words when we explored New York City together: "Listen when the city speaks and follow where it leads."

We satisfied our late-night cravings with homemade ice cream sandwiched between Toll House cookies so fresh the chocolate chips were still gooey. There is something about sharing food with a lover. Eating the sides up to the middle and negotiating the last bite, do you let him have it? Does he insist that you do? Do you feed it to him on the spoon? I picked up the messy, final morsel and placed it on his tongue. He swallowed and licked my sticky fingers, giving me shivers.

Dennis and I kept in touch, ever plotting our next get-together, and I scoured my workload for a trip where we could connect. We kept our new relationship energy fueled with texting, but I had no expectations other than getting together when logistics allowed. While I would have liked to see Dennis more often, the elusive nature of our rendezvous made them even more exciting. His sexy and thoughtful, if sporadic, "thinking of you" texts always made me smile. I looked forward to each meeting with him and to seeing Violet when possible. She was supportive of our relationship, telling me, "I compersion hard when Dennis connects with someone." I liked that. *Compersion* as a verb.

When Dennis and I met at kinky summer camp and he told me he was mesmerized by my luscious breasts—oh, and my snarky wit—I figured what happened at kinky camp would stay there. I did not envision that we would so easily connect on business trips, trading stories, learning the curves and reactions of each other's bodies, and playfully, semi-sadistically, teasing those bodies to the verge of release.

I treasured the times we occupied our two-person sphere for a night or two after our workdays were done. Then we smiled our farewells until our paths crossed again. I loved the way his eyes blinked at me when he smiled. I laughed at his dad jokes and puns, but I was realistic. We lived half a country apart. I figured we could enjoy each other's company when the planets aligned because what else could we be but comets?

Less than a year after we met at summer camp, Dennis changed jobs. He would be moving to my neighborhood. I volunteered to be his plus-one to check out prospective apartments for him, Violet, Zoey, and their pets. I showed him the dog park and my favorite pho restaurant.

After one of those apartment visits, I paused to check in with Dennis. He and his crew would be living half a mile from me and Eric. With only one traffic light between us, how would our new proximity affect what had been a low expectation dynamic? Maybe Dennis's priorities would keep us casual partners, or maybe we would see each other more regularly. I could manage my expectations if I had information—a priceless commodity. In my experience, unrealistic, unmet, and *uncommunicated* expectations paved the road to breakdowns and breakups.

"Dennis," I began, "what are you thinking about seeing me after you move here?"

"I definitely want to see you," Dennis beamed. "Neighbor." He winked.

I felt a flutter of joy, but I waited for him to expand, not wanting to presume anything. When I had met Violet, now Dennis's wife, a year before, I had perceived no danger vibes, but that seemed like a lifetime ago. Being her husband's occasional out-of-town partner was one thing; living within shouting distance was another.

"I was thinking that we could get together about every ten days to two weeks, if that works for you," Dennis said.

I smiled. "Sounds good." Between work and my other commitments, that frequency seemed just right.

Over the next two years, Dennis and his household became beloved members of the polycule I shared with Eric and our other partners. Eric, as was his poly style, man-crushed on his metamour. He was forever reminding me what a great guy Dennis was, as ready to help us set up the house for an epic dance party as he was to solve my IT issues or engage in the kitchen table polyamory Eric enjoyed, as distinguished from *parallel polyamory*, where relationships were kept separate.

Eric was right. Dennis was a great guy. Our connection was easy and comfortable while being sexy and fun. Violet turned out to be an easygoing metamour. We developed a friendship over coffee and kvetching. I saw what Dennis loved about her. Eric was smitten with her, too. Eric and Violet—both extroverts—teased Dennis and me about our D&D evenings at home—shorthand for Dinner and Dystopia—when we ate takeout and watched *The Handmaid's Tale*.

On our third campiversary, Dennis and I were enjoying after-sex solitude under the stars, grinning at each other like two goofy kids with a secret. Looking into Dennis's clear gray eyes, framed with enviably long lashes, I felt content and achingly close to him. I felt safe saying, for the first time in our relationship, "You know, I love you."

Dennis gave me a smile that warmed me from the inside out.

"I love you and Eric," he said.

My smile froze on my face as my thoughts raced. *Aw, that's nice that he loves my husband and me, um, as a unit, but wait, that's, well, I mean . . . ?*

I tried not to get hung up on the inclusion of Eric. *Dennis and I cared about each other, and that was good. I wanted to be able to express how I felt so I did. That was also good.*

Still . . . the words "I love you" continued to be the square peg in the round hole of all my relationships except the one I had with Eric. Hank had said,

"Maybe I only have enough love in my heart for Sylvia," the wife he divorced two years later. "I care about you. Isn't that the same thing anyway?" he had said.

I won't make the mistake of saying that again, I vowed, and my next poly relationship with Lee suffered for it.

I finally said it to Wesley when we had been dating for two years. After emerging from a workshop at a poly conference on vulnerability, a class that left me uncharacteristically tearful, I told Wesley that I wanted to be free to express my feelings. As a result of Hank's reaction years earlier, I had shut that down. I was trying to take chances with my heart.

Wesley, whom I had met six months before I met Dennis, squeezed my hand.

He said, "Oh, thank you, Natalie. That's so nice. I care about you very much, too. I am not going to say it back because I am trying not to say that so much." He told me that his local partner, Piper, said "I love you" so often and expected so much that he was being more parsimonious with the expression. *For fuck's sake times two.*

"I understand," I said, trying to.

Wesley and Piper broke up not long after our exchange. He traded "I love yous" within weeks of dating a new, local girlfriend. Wesley joyfully shared the news with me, his long-distance partner. I messaged, "How nice!" Texting hid my clenched jaw.

After almost ten years of navigating long-term poly relationships—with Hank, Lee, Wesley, and Dennis—I rationalized: *Eric loves me, and I love him. That's more than many people have. I should be thankful. Eric and his girlfriends exchange "I love yous" with abandon, but maybe that is not my polyamorous lot. Polyfuckery for me, then! I guess I am just not that lovable to anyone but Eric. Stable, smart, sexy—but not someone you fall in love with.*

Breathing now. I was fine. Fine. But also, fuck you, romantic societal norms that weighed down three damn words with so much import and emotion.

If I seem hung up—just a skosh—on this perilous love juncture in a relationship, given my poly experiences, you may understand. Dennis, however, did not know. He did not know that I feared that the only love relationship that I, a poly*amorous* woman, would ever have would be with my husband. I had not told Dennis about Hank or Lee or Wesley. I couldn't blame him for not knowing, so I didn't.

There was a lot I didn't know about Dennis's attachment history and relationships, and I took a measured approach to asking. I assumed his wife was the one he talked to about that, just as Eric was my go-to person for unloading emotional baggage. Dennis and I cared about each other. Undoubtedly, we would rescue each other from a broken-down car on the side of the road, but we would not be each other's first call. That would be our spouses. We were in harmony there.

I had thought we were of the same mind about what we felt for each other. I figured what Dennis said that night under the stars was what he was able to say, so I let it be. Nothing changed between us. We continued to see each other. We continued to care about each other. Our polycule became closer, sharing holidays, birthdays, and movie nights.

During one of our text chats more than a year after that campiversary exchange, without overthinking it, I messaged Dennis that I loved him while we were saying warm things to each other. He texted back "I love you and Eric" and added a kissy face.

I laughed. I knew he and Eric had mutual crushes—that was adorable—*but Dennis,* I thought, *that's not what I meant when I said I loved you, and I know you know that.*

The next time it happened—yes, a third time—I finally called him on it.

"Dennis, just so you know, nothing will change between us if you say you love me without including Eric. I will not expect anything more from you." I am sure I added some silly emoticon for laughing.

Almost immediately, Dennis texted back, "I love you."

Can you guess what happened?

Nothing. Nothing changed except we started saying it face to face—can you believe such daring? The sky did not fall. I did not demand to see him more often. We did not devolve into jealousy and bickering. We did not leave our spouses.

We became more open and caring with each other. I asked more about what was going on in his heart and in his head. He shared what he felt comfortable sharing, and his confiding in me brought us closer. We supported each other in ways we would have previously reserved for our spouses. We offered each other additional shoulders to spread the burden and the care.

That is the dividend of polyamory—more partners mean more hugs to hold you, more brains to problem-solve, and more love to remind you how lucky you are to be alive.

24.
Thanksgiving

"Mom, who are all these people?" Will had asked, bending his lean frame down to me.

I had looked up from stirring gravy and wiped my hands on my apron. Two long folding tables, set for sixteen, stood end to end in the living room. Two eight-year-olds ran between the furniture, and one short-haired dog was underfoot.

That was last year. Maybe I had gone overboard. Then came my mom guilt. I had told myself I would curb my enthusiasm this Thanksgiving while Will was home from college. But I found it hard to turn away anyone. *What's just one more?* I kept thinking.

Thanksgiving was my favorite holiday—the day I made Mom's sweeter-than-candy sweet potato casserole and my mother-in-law's chocolate meringue pie. It was the day I employed my cousin's trick for moist turkey—two quarts of chicken broth in the roasting pan. Out came our wedding china, Mom's oh-my-god-be-careful I-had-them-shipped-from-Ireland Waterford crystal wine stems and water goblets, and my grandmother's Depression-era silverware, stored in a tarnish-protecting, fabric-lined wooden box. Mini gourds and fresh flowers adorned the table. Eric calligraphed the names of each guest on place cards. As my Aunt Sarah would say, we did the whole schmear.

This Thanksgiving I had vowed to go small. Just family. But in mid-November, when I pictured our table of three, it just seemed, well, sad. Mom, Dad, and Teenager with sometimes introverted moods seemed not enough. We didn't even have a buffer.

I texted Dennis. He, Violet, Zoey, and Violet's boyfriend, Eddie, had become part of our poly family, and Thanksgiving was for family after all.

"Hey, cutie. What are your Thanksgiving plans?" I asked Dennis.

Dennis responded, "We aren't doing anything specific, but we are staying in town."

"Want to join us?"

"We'd love to! What can I cook or bring?"

I thought about the dishes I planned to make. "Let me think about that."

"Sure," Dennis responded and then added, "Can we wear pajamas to dinner?"

I stifled a laugh as I reread the text. "Sure, as long as you shower first."

On Thanksgiving, I woke early to bake the chocolate pie and prep the turkey for roasting. I was on Day Four of my Holiday Plan. Eric teased me about my multi-day, multi-step strategy. My typed chart listing the prep and cooking or baking time of all dishes and the varied oven temperatures was held to the fridge door by three magnets. Adding tick marks next to each completed task was my reward.

Dennis had offered to come over and help on Wednesday night or early on Thursday.

"I can cook, you know," he said. "Or chop or just keep you company."

"That's very sweet, but no, thank you. I have a plan," I said.

"Trust me, brother," said Eric. "Give Natalie room to make her magic. Those who get in her way might get stepped on, not necessarily on purpose, but she does wield the carving knife, and the ER on Thanksgiving is a zoo. I would prefer to avoid it."

Eric set out his place cards with me at the head of the table.

"No, wait, that's always your seat. I sit here, on the side near the kitchen for quick access," I said, about to move the card.

"Natalie, you did all the work," he said. "You should sit there."

I examined the seating arrangement. Eric was on my right. Dennis was on my left. Violet was next to her husband, and her boyfriend Eddie was on her left. Across the table from Eddie was Zoey, then our son, Will, next to his father. The seating made sense. We were a respectable seven-head count.

My polycule mates were on time at two-thirty. I credited Violet for her timely herding of the crew. Tardiness irritated her. *Thank you, metamour, for not adding to my hostess stress.* Dennis cooked a massive pot of truffle mashed potatoes. Zoey made pumpkin cheesecake. Both were delicious. No one wore pajamas.

We served buffet style, eating leisurely and talking easily. Will comfortably participated in the conversation, so comfortably that I heard a few curse words. I refrained from parental chiding and just listened with affection to my dear ones enjoying the family meal.

Will had met Dennis a few times at the house. Will was studying computer science, and Dennis was an IT savant, so I figured their shared interest would grease the wheels. He and Zoey worked together doing computer genius stuff I could not pretend to understand, but Dennis had an approachable way of explaining that my liberal arts brain appreciated. Violet was a gaming whiz, so everyone, except me and Eric, geeked on gaming. She and her partners were in the process of painting and prepping her dungeon space to re-up her pro-domme business. Eddie, currently working a retail job while he looked for a tech position, was about seven years older than Will. Dennis, Violet, and Zoey were all in their early thirties. Violet and Will shared a birth date, a connection that touched me in a way I could not quite explain.

For dessert, Zoey's creamy cheesecake was a hit. "Hey, Mom, can you get the recipe?" Will asked me between gulps.

We chatted and lounged on the sofas, watching funny YouTube videos, movie trailers, and *Saturday Night Live* clips. We had round two of turkey and trimmings and, after more hanging out, were startled to realize that it was eleven o'clock. I tossed Will my car keys, and he drove Dennis and the crew to their apartment, five minutes away.

Violet later told me that on the drive home, Will said, "You guys are not like my parents' extrovert friends. I didn't want to go upstairs to my room." I think that was my son's way of saying that he had a good Thanksgiving.

EPILOGUE

If I could talk to my younger self, I wonder what I would tell her about polyamory—and whether I would be wasting my breath.

As a parent, I realize that there are some things your children will not hear, no matter how often or pointedly you say them. It's as if their ear canals haven't formed well enough to receive sound, so they are unable to hear you warn them off ill-advised behavior like procrastinating on a semester-long project or driving thirty hours without a bathroom break. Some things we have to figure out for ourselves.

When I don my hopeful hat, I imagine having a savvy girlfriend or an enlightened aunt clue me in about polyamory. Maybe Eric and I could have explored this path together sooner, before his infidelity. I think about Bennett, the young writer who knew from adolescence that dating one girl at a time didn't make sense to him.

I think about Eric, who seemed to find his true self when he found polyamory. If he had been poly or known he was when I met him, would we have dated and fallen in love? Doubtful. If you had asked me to spell non-monogamy—I am still not sure whether to use a hyphen—much less engage in it, it would have been like suggesting we eat pie underwater. Who would *want* to do that? The younger me was inexperienced at even monogamous relationships. The notion of entering a multifaceted romance might very well have shocked my naïve self toward a nunnery.

As a child, I dressed like my peers and tuned the radio to the Top 40 station. I listened to my parents to such an extent that they trusted me not to have a curfew. That seems uncool to admit.

I can't picture myself ever suggesting consensual non-monogamy. I only considered it when Eric inserted the idea into our marriage. It originally went over like a lead balloon, but to my surprise, it eventually took flight. If Eric had suggested we have an open relationship when we were in college—the term *polyamory* had not been coined yet—I probably would have walked away. I knew nothing about consensual non-monogamous relationships. I had a passing familiarity with the *polygamy* of Mormon fundamentalists, but I gave little thought to the marriage of one man to multiple women, dismissing it as a religious patriarchal peculiarity that could easily be abusive.

In the introduction to this book, I may have come across as starry-eyed by saying that polyamory changed my life. Yes, it did. Many events affected me to varying degrees—falling in love with Eric, my first jury trial, becoming a parent, cancer, cooking without a recipe, discovering the ache and bliss of solo bike rides, the death of my parents, and infidelity in my marriage. I had to experience them to understand them; to discover or survive them.

To say that polyamory not only opened up my marriage but also opened up my life is not an exaggeration. The life skills I developed to examine and ultimately embrace polyamory were skills that also mellowed my harshness, lessened my judgments, taught me patience and tolerance, and allowed me to unclench my fist and offer my hand. When I think of all the people I have met—some crazy and unbalanced, some affectionate and tolerant, and some all those things at once—and how I might have spent the rest of my days not experiencing life with them and through them, I ache with knowing how much I would have lost.

For me, polyamory is not the end. It is the means. It is how life offered me a new pair of glasses. A childhood friend told me that when she got her first pair of glasses, she looked up at the trees in her yard. She was awed to see individual leaves and upset that she had been blind to what had always been visible to others.

Only upon looking back do I see how static and trapped I was in my objectively successful life with my husband, child, career, house, and dog. There were community activities, family we loved, and, more often than not, enough money. There was also a husband who, despite his love for me, was unhappy with the confines of our traditional domestication. I did not understand that until the cheating started.

If I could tell my younger self something and make it stick, I would tell her to loosen up and consider life outside the box you think you know. I smile at my treasure trove of discoveries because I said yes to polyamory.

On my deathbed, I want to say yes, I did all the things, loved all the people and let them know it, and suffered and shared and grew and tried and failed. Felix was part of that journey. I do not regret what we went through. I do not regret Hank or Lee or Trevor or Bennett or the surgical resident who fell asleep on me or the guy that Eric pulled off me at a swinger party because he thought he was too much of a jerk to bed his wife.

Eric is woven into my narrative like a hammock into which I can climb, do acrobatics, or just rest my head. His patience, guidance, and relative sanity form a backdrop to my non-monogamous journey. His level voice is the narrator in my head, reminding me to take a breath when I expect too much of myself or others or when I am more closed off than open. His ability to jump in where I draw back could startle my more reticent self, but it allowed me to engage—or not—in smaller or larger ways, depending on my choice.

I am grateful to Eric for showing me an open door. A part of me was angry with him for a long time. His cheating led me to doubt his love and to doubt myself. I finally realized that his infidelity was not solely about me, and that not everything that happens during a marriage or any long-term relationship is about that relationship.

That Eric shared his journey with me, and not in spite of or without me, was a gift. He could have walked away. He could have presumed that non-monogamy would be a deal-breaker, marriage ender, or divorce starter. It was not easy to tell me that he wanted something else, something more, something so different than what we had been taught to even consider, much less embrace.

Every day, Eric and I navigate our lives. Most of it is the same as anyone—work, family, household chores, medical appointments, celebrations, and disappointments. I am not saying we don't bicker about bills, schedules, politics, and emotions. There are times when I snipe, or he seethes, or vice versa. There is envy and impatience and a lack of sympathy because we are human, and we feel and think, hurt and love.

We talk so much. We touch. We tell each other we love and value each other because we do and because it is important to make it heard. For a long time, I wondered if my polyamory was limited to polyfuckery, whether I would say "I love you" to anyone but Eric, and they would say it back, but I know now that my heart is wide and deep and caring. As to how resilient it is, I am still finding out.

* * *

I met Pete the summer I borrowed the apartment of an absent snowbird for a few days after a work trip to South Florida. I found solitude on the sunlit beach in the mornings and wrote during the rainy afternoons. A slender, short, dark-featured artist, Pete was the most introverted young man I had dated. He had small, silver snakebite rings that pierced both sides of his lower lip, which he absently fingered as I imagined someone with a handlebar mustache would.

I had thought he was several years younger than his thirty-three years because his quiet and deliberate manner came across as hesitant and boyish. He liked to talk to me about polyamory, and I liked to hear how he navigated his dating life. Pete used the term *polyamorous*, not the shorthand *poly*, which was my default, and I noticed. He said it in a way that gave import to the term, as if he was invoking something consequential, in a way a mother might call her son by his full name when she wanted his undivided attention.

When I met him, Pete was dating two women in their early twenties who were new to polyamory and navigating metamour-to-metamour dynamics. When one of Pete's girlfriends finally met the other, after several months of being metamours, she could not overcome her jealousy, and she and Pete broke up. Pete had been the hinge between two women who were seeing only him—a mono-poly-mono V. I was sympathetic that his partners could not find a way to get along as two people who cared about Pete rather than as members of opposing teams vying for a prize.

The following summer, I met Pete for dinner after my trial concluded.

"I'd like to show you the beach at night, if you'd like to go," he said tentatively. "I know a good spot."

"Lead on," I said.

It was past eleven, and the night was dark. After I parked the rental car, I baby-stepped along a path leading from the road to the sand. The moon, at its zenith, lit our way. We were completely alone.

We settled onto the sand, having no towels on our impromptu visit. Propped on my elbows, butt on the beach, I dug canals with my bare heels, finding the coolness beneath the warm sand. I was calmed by the rhythmic ebb and flow of the sea and the sable shroud of the sky. As I gazed out toward the black ocean, I could see little more than the shimmer of moonlight on the cusp of the gentle waves.

We were staring silently at the water when Pete said, "I just noticed that big rock. Did you see it before?"

I turned my head a fraction to where he was looking and saw a large, dark, round shape, like a mound of sand. I shook my head. "No, that's weird." Then, startled, I scooted back a few paces like a crab and said, "I think it moved."

Pete stood up halfway to a crouching position, peering ahead. "That's a sea turtle. We have to leave," he whispered as he stood up. "She's coming ashore to lay her eggs. They're easily frightened by motion or light. If we interrupt her, she may get spooked and retreat to the ocean with a belly full of eggs, which can be deadly."

I reached for my shoes, and when I looked back at the black orb on the sand, it had moved up the beach closer to us. It was huge. It seemed like a monster creeping out from the sea. I couldn't make out its features because it was so dark. We backed away as quietly as possible.

We were a third of the way down the narrow, sandy path from the beach to the road when my hands touched my ears in a reflexive check for my silver hoop earrings. I stopped walking and told Pete to wait.

He turned to face me. "What's up?"

I said, "I lost an earring in the sand."

"Do you want to go back for it?"

I hesitated. I would have let it go, but the earrings had been a birthday present from Will. The needle in a haystack adage came to mind, but I had to look for it. If the earring had dropped and not been buried, we might have a chance. The ridges in the beach where my heels had disturbed the sand were easy markers for Pete's sharp eyes. The earring was lying atop the sand, and Pete scooped it up.

We watched the turtle continue her slow and steady advance up the beach for a spot to start her flippers pushing away the sand to make her nest, and we began our retreat once again. I saw that a couple had wandered along the shoreline, taken out their phones with the bright screen lights, and were snapping photos of the turtle.

"No," I whisper-shouted to them, trying not to disturb the mama turtle while waving my arms to get their attention. "You'll scare her away," I said.

They either didn't hear or didn't care because they continued to flash their phones at the turtle. I was beside myself, attempting to ward them off without shouting and spooking the turtle. Sadly, but predictably, the sea turtle retreated to the water without laying her eggs. I held on to the hope that the mama turtle would come ashore again the following moonlit night, as Pete said could happen.

Pete and I picked our way along the dark path to the car, and my eyes could not help but follow the moon. I felt aglow, like a silent witness to a mystical, albeit aborted, ceremony. I took Pete's hand and thanked him. As was his way, Pete nodded once and strolled on.

If I were monogamous, that night would not have happened. I would not have met Pete on a dating site because monogamous married people don't date. Even if I had met him in a socially acceptable context, such as a work conference, it would have been the fuel of gossip for the two of us to head to the beach alone in the black of night to contemplate the stars because married women don't do that with single men. We would not have shared the sacred space that the nocturnal shore offered. I would not have been privy to the magic of nature and the cycle of the sea. I hold that evening close to my breast, a cherished moment.

When I see an exceptionally brilliant moon suspended in a pitch sky, I think of that night and of all the ways that polyamory has enhanced my life and helped me strive to be a better person. Eventually, I float back to the ground and face myself. I may like myself more, but I still have miles to go, some of it uphill. I am more open, loving, inquisitive, and interactive. I am more fulfilled. I believe in the polyamorous path I have chosen because I did ultimately choose it.

At times, I am jealous, needy, impatient, selfish, and intolerant, but who I am is neither the blame nor the acquittal of polyamory. Engaging in polyamory enabled growth. It gave me permission to explore outside the confines of what I knew as the monogamous narrative. It offered me options I did not know existed, options I could reject, accept, or tailor for the best fit.

That I am an unfinished work is not a cliché to me. I am not unquestionably resolved until my hands lie, finally, folded on my chest. Until then, I am invigorated by the prospect of all I will experience and learn and all the people I have yet to meet as I live my polyamorous life.

Acknowledgments

To those who supported me on my journey to commit to bits and bytes the story of my polyamorous life, I offer my sincere thanks. At long last, I can delete the section in my will that divulges my laptop password and implores my loved ones to give life to an especially large Word file.

KC, did you ever imagine our trading story-length emails would morph into this?

TS, you heard my five-minute monologue at an open mic night and invited me into a group of real writers; your edits and commentary gave me valuable perspective.

Cat, you suggested we co-work at the library to keep me on task. You only showed up once—girl!—but I kept going back.

The Central Library, whose Quiet Room melted distractions; the Authors Guild, for access to contracting language and fulsome commentary, an indispensable resource for navigating and negotiating a publishing contract.

Daniela at Skyhorse, who believed in this book; Rachael, who provided a platform on Medium to share my stories; TD, for honest edits and unshakable cheerleading.

My sister, GK, ESN, and PK, for listening to my processing and reading my work; Fiona, Rae, and Trisha, my ride-or-die; Cunning Minx and Lusty Guy, whose podcast advice made me feel less alone; Dennis, my D&D partner and so much more.

Zella, whose savvy and indispensable editorial scalpel was bathed in more love than blood.

My son, who challenges me and lifts me higher.

My husband, who said, after I came home with tales from yet another first date, "You know, you should write a book."